Menopause, Naturally

PREPARING FOR THE SECOND HALF OF LIFE

REVISED EDITION

Sadja Greenwood, M.D.

Illustrations by Marcia Quackenbush

VOLCANO PRESS

Volcano, California

 PRINTED ON RECYCLED PAPER

Library of Congress Cataloging in Publication Data

Greenwood, Sadja, 1930–
    Menopause, naturally.

    Bibliography: p.
    1. Menopause.   2. Middle aged women—Health and hygiene.
I. Title.
RG186.G74   1989   618.1'75   88–202
ISBN 0-912078-83-9

Volcano Press participates in the Cataloging in Publication Program of the Library of Congress. However, in our opinion, the data provided us for this book by CIP does not adequately nor accurately reflect its scope and content. Therefore, we are offering our librarian/users the choice between LC's treatment and an Alternative CIP prepared by Sanford Berman, Head Cataloger at Hennepin County Library, Edina, Minnesota.

Library of Congress Cataloging in Publication Data

Greenwood, Sadja, 1930–
    Menopause, naturally. Revised: preparing for the second half of life.
Volcano Press, Volcano, CA, copyright 1984, 1989.
    PARTIAL CONTENTS: Sex in the second half of life.   –Keep your bones strong—how to avoid osteoporosis.   –When periods stop before 40.   –Estrogen replacement therapy: the pros, cons, and unkowns.   –Beliefs about aging.   –Relaxation: calming down and letting go.   –Use it or lose it: exercise in mid-life.
    1. Menopause.   2. Middle aged women—Health.
3. Osteoporosis—Prevention.   4. Middle aged women—Sexuality.   5. Holistic health.   6. Exercise for middle aged persons.   7. Estrogen replacement therapy.   8. Relaxation.
I. Title.
    II. Volcano Press.   III. Title: Naturally, menopause.
                  618.175

Production Coordination, Book and Cover Design: Marie Carluccio
Composition: Sunflower, Compositærs
Typography: Access Typography

Printed in the United States of America.

10 9 8 7 6 5 4 3 2

Volcano Press
P.O. Box 270
Volcano, CA 95689
Tel: (209) 296-3445
Telex: 650-3491755
Fax: (209) 296-4515

CONTENTS

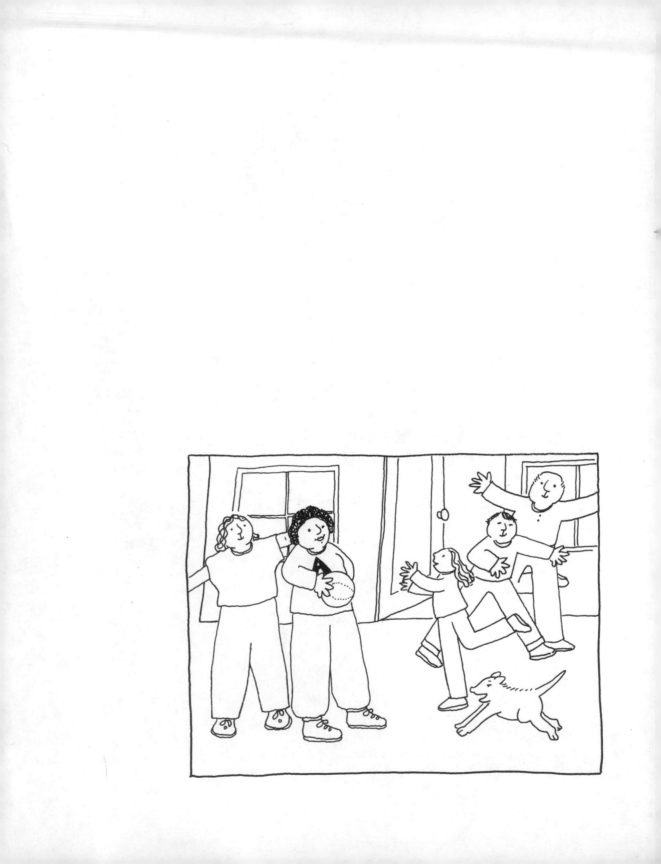

Author's Preface

My own menopause put me in awe of the human body. I marveled at the way that the process of fertility, beginning around age 13, follows nature's plan and comes to a predictable close about 37 years later. I wanted to know more about these intricate mechanisms and lifetime purposes of our bodies, and how we could get in harmony with our changes.

These questions led me to set up a mid-life and menopause service in a local women's clinic. I was struck by the complexity and diversity of each woman's menopausal experiences, and began to write guidelines for ways to stay healthy in mid-life, emphasizing nutrition and enjoyable exercise. I realized that an individual approach to hormone use was also clearly necessary — but relatively complex. As I worked on these questions, the publisher and editor of Volcano Press suggested that I expand my guidelines into a book. This idea seemed absolutely right to me and the process began.

I am a general practice physician with a major interest in gynecology and women's health care, and an assistant clinical professor in the Department of Obstetrics, Gynecology, and Reproductive Sciences at the University of California Medical Center, San Francisco.

After practicing in a fairly traditional way for many years, and feeling perpetually stressed by the competing needs of work and raising children, I developed an illness that made me slow down and reassess my life. A patient for the first time, I understood the fear of disease, the power of modern medical treatment, and the awesome side effects they create. My reaction was to try my utmost to get healthy and stay that way. I explored the values of nutrition, exercise, relaxation, meditation, imagery, and hope and humor, and found that a great deal being written on these subjects is of relevance to the prevention and cure of disease. I also discovered that exciting and scientifically sound papers that speak about prevention are buried in specialist medical journals, where they are largely ignored. We doctors are so busy diagnosing and treating illness that we have no time to teach ourselves or our patients how to stay well.

I decided to change my own life in a healthier direction, and to introduce more basic teachings about nutrition, relaxation, and physical activity into my medical practice. After all, the word "doctor" comes from the Latin word for teacher. I see this book on the menopause as an outgrowth of this process — an integration of my work with mid-life women and my interests in the promotion of health.

So there you have it. I am a 57-year-old doctor, mother of two grown sons, a vegetarian, and a hiker, looking for the truths about life and the joy in every day.

In this updated edition of *Menopause, Naturally* I have carefully assessed the changes in scientific knowledge since the book first came out in 1984. There is new material on the treatment of uterine fibroids without hysterectomy, ovarian function with aging, the mechanisms and treatment of hot flashes, and on osteoporosis and calcium intake. I share the latest information on the lowest effective dose of estrogen, the estrogen "patch," and the risks and benefits of estrogen replacement therapy. Risk factors for breast cancer are updated. The nutrition section contains a new emphasis on the benefits of fish and olive oil, and the negative effects of artificial sweeteners.

I want to acknowledge the many people who have helped me with this book. First and foremost Ruth Gottstein, the publisher and editor of Volcano Press, and her colleagues Leigh Davidson and Marie Carluccio — these three women have been incredibly supportive and helpful every step of the way. The wonderful drawings of Marcia Quackenbush inspire me to see the essence of people and the glow and humor in life. My companion, Alan Margolis, has given me unfailing encouragement and discerning suggestions from his extensive gynecologic background.

I want to thank the following physicians and scientists for their help, through their published work and via telephone calls: Bruce Ettinger, Robert Heaney, Phillip Hoffman, Morris Notelovitz, Diana Petitti, and Everett Smith. Thanks also to Dr. Ron Ruggiero for his great help in the area of pharmacology. Another thank you goes to those who read and critiqued the book in its various stages — Joani Blank, Sally Campbell, Mary Davies, Neshama Franklin, Vicki Lansky, and Joan Robbins.

I also appreciate the excellent work of Peggi Oakley of Sunflower, Compositærs, in preparing the manuscript. The medical library at the University of California Medical Center in San Francisco, and the people who work there, are an extremely valuable scientific resource.

I also want to thank my mother for the inspiration of her example — she has more zest after the menopause than most of us have in a lifetime; she showed me the positives and strengths of being a woman.

Finally, I must acknowledge the importance of my patients, especially those in the second half of life, for showing me the many facets of human experience and the need for an individualized approach to medical treatment.

Sadja Greenwood, M.D., M.P.H.
San Francisco, California
June 1988

"The most creative force in the world is the menopausal woman with zest."

—MARGARET MEAD

We are not troubled by things, but by the opinions which we have of things.

— Epictetus

Cecilia walked rapidly into my office and pulled out her notes. "Look at this record of my periods," she said with despair. "I'm probably going through the menopause at 42. It's ironic that I'll fall apart at a time when I've finally found the right job and a good relationship." After listening to Cecilia and examining her, I explained to her that her frequent heavier periods were not a sign of the menopause, but might be related to a small fibroid tumor on her uterus, or to her increasing use of alcohol to calm herself after long hours of exacting work. I found that she considered the menopause to be a tragic time in life because of vivid memories of her mother's problems after having a hysterectomy at age 40. Her mother's regrets over this surgical menopause had greatly influenced Cecilia's early life.

Later in the same day Paula was telling me about her intense feelings of irritability and depression before her periods. "Is this what it's like to go through the menopause?" she asked. "If so, I'm really dreading it."

Menopause: Fallacies, Facts, and New Possibilities

Neither of these women was actually going through the menopause, but both showed me that they needed information and a more positive view about this natural transition between the years of fertility and the second half of life. Negative messages about menopause abound in our culture — in cartoons, "old wives' tales," and medical texts. Fear and dread of the "change of life" are easy to acquire and can influence our behavior, our beliefs, and our bodies in subtly destructive ways.

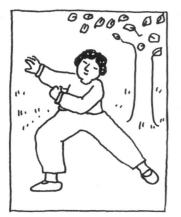

Lillian, a Chinese-American woman of 50, viewed her menopause more positively. Her periods had stopped in her late 40s. Lillian said, "Getting rid of my periods was such a relief to me. I feel very balanced now. I took up Tai Chi about 10 years ago because I was getting sluggish, and that has made a big difference in my life. I do it every morning before work." Listening to Lillian made me reflect that she came from a culture with more respect for aging. She had also found a daily exercise that increased her strength and her feelings of inner harmony. Her menopause had been a smooth transition.

As a physician, I am always gathering information about the way people lead their daily lives and the way they feel about themselves. I have found that women who enter the menopause viewing it as a natural process or transition have an easier time than those who view it as a crisis. Women who exercise daily, eat healthy food, and work on achieving emotional balance usually manage to avoid many of the ills of mid-life. Moreover, adopting such practices can cure many problems more reliably than drugs or surgery. Skillful physicians can help their patients decide when counseling and lifestyle changes are sufficient, or when medicine or life-saving technology is needed.

In recent years I have conducted a special clinic for mid-life women and have taken part in numerous discussion groups on the menopause. I have been impressed by the help that women

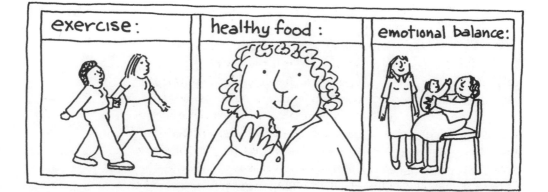

exercise: healthy food: emotional balance:

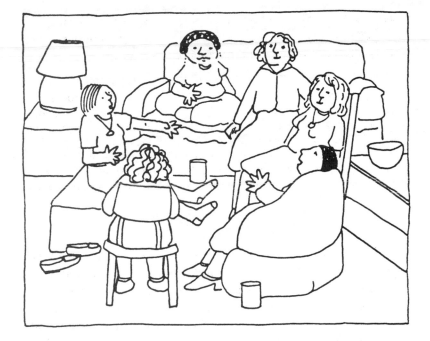

can give to each other in open discussions, and by the power of accurate, nonthreatening information.

What *does* happen in the menopause? Strictly speaking, the word "menopause" refers only to the final menstrual period. In common usage, however, it designates a transitional time from a few years before the last menses to a year after it. As hormone output from the ovaries declines, menstrual periods become irregular and then disappear. Symptoms such as hot flashes, night sweats, and vaginal dryness are experienced at this time by four out of five women. The menopause usually occurs between 48 and 52, but it often happens earlier and occasionally later.

We don't know why the menopause occurs in human beings but not in animals. Anthropologists have suggested that the menopause has benefited our species during evolution, by releasing women from the stresses and dangers of childbearing to raise their late-born children and transmit cultural knowledge. They also point out that the menopausal transition is viewed very differently from one society to another. In Western culture, with its strong emphasis on female youth and beauty, the menopause is seen as a time of decline and loss of status for women. Belief in "progress" and in the taming and changing of natural forces

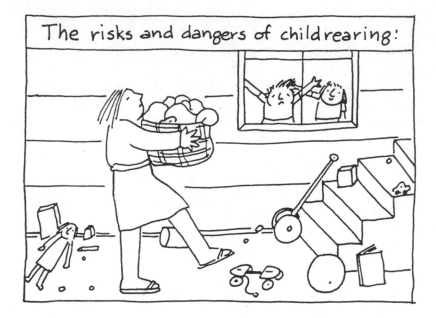

The risks and dangers of childrearing:

makes us willing to alter women's hormonal levels in mid-life. The menopause is viewed as a medical event — even a disease process — which requires treatment and careful medical follow-up. Other societies see the menopause very differently. Among many non-Western groups, the older woman enjoys increased status in the family and greater freedom in society at large. Menopause and the cessation of childbearing become positive events in a woman's life, and physical symptoms are given less attention.

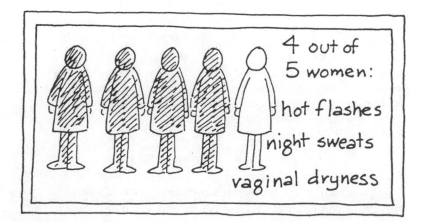

4 out of 5 women:

hot flashes

night sweats

vaginal dryness

Since the 1960s, profound changes have occurred in women's perceptions of their rights and roles in our society. Women are more active in every phase of community life, and more aware of their own needs and directions. This development has been linked to momentous changes in women's health care, including the ability to choose when or whether to have children, and a driving need on the part of many women to understand their bodies and participate in decisions about their own health or illness. Today, as millions of women reach their 40s and 50s they are seeking new approaches to the menopause. They want to replace the negative stereotypes of the menopausal woman with a realistic and positive outlook. This new viewpoint will flourish as women learn more about how to live through the changes of middle age with maximum health and equanimity.

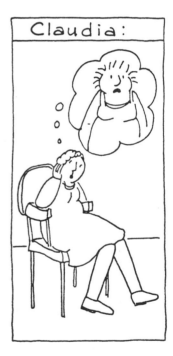

"You mean I don't have to go crazy in the menopause?" Claudia laughed at herself as she asked this question, but there was an edge of fear in her voice. "Whenever I think of my mother and her depressions I get really worried." When she analyzed it, Claudia wasn't so sure that her mother was more depressed in the menopause than she had been years earlier or later. However, she had heard other relatives blame her mother's condition on "the change of life" and had accepted this explanation. Years later, as she approached the menopause herself, she found that she had an irrational dread of reliving her mother's example. An open discussion and explanation of the menopause helped her to see her own future as different from her mother's.

Belle looked like she had a lot to say, and I listened intently to her story. "At first the menopause was very difficult for me. I was waking at night with hot flashes and couldn't get back to sleep. I felt very self-conscious at work whenever I had one. My daughter was driving me nuts, which didn't help. My doctor said I should take estrogen pills, but they made my breasts extremely sore and gave me a funny feeling in my head. Then a friend of mine at work started taking me to her yoga class. That really turned things around for me. I guess I learned how to relax for the first time in my life. My body felt better; I stopped the estrogen and started vitamins. The hot flashes still come but they don't bother me any more. I've learned so much in that class that I think I feel healthier than when I was 30." Belle did a yoga posture to show me how supple she had become. I was also impressed that her blood pressure was low and her heart rate slow and even.

I have two major aims in this book — to provide as much information as possible on how to promote good health and avoid illness in the second half of life, and to discuss interesting and controversial questions about the menopause — such as why bleeding is irregular and hot flashes occur, how to deal with vaginal soreness, how to make an informed decision about estrogen use, and how to avoid brittle bones (osteoporosis).

Margaret Mead, the well-known anthropologist, spoke about post-menopausal zest, or PMZ. I've seen women who have PMZ and those who don't, and those who find it after a long process of self-exploration and self-healing. Perhaps I can show you some short cuts along the way.

"One month I can hardly get out of the house because of the bleeding I'm having, and the next month there's almost nothing. I never know what to expect these days."

"My periods are getting closer together and sometimes they are really heavy. Is that normal at 48?"

"Last month my period didn't come at all. I started waking up at night feeling really hot, and I couldn't get back to sleep. Then I had another period and everything is back to normal."

"My husband died when I was 49. It was a terrible time. I never had another period after his death, but I never had any menopausal symptoms either."

The Hows and Whys of Menopausal Bleeding

All these and many other patterns can occur in the menopause. Let's review what is known about menstruation and its somewhat erratic behavior at this time of life. As the illustration shows, the uterus is a pear-shaped organ that develops a lining of cells and blood vessels every month in the fertile years. A menstrual period occurs when the uterus sheds this lining. This happens at regular intervals to most women under 45.

Each month the ovaries produce the hormones estrogen and progesterone in a predictable pattern. Estrogen is produced in the first half of the cycle in increasing amounts, causing a thick lining to grow in the uterus. At mid-cycle one ovary produces a mature egg cell, or ovum, which travels down a narrow tube into the uterus. This event is called ovulation, and marks the time when pregnancy can occur. After ovulation, in the 2 weeks before the next menstrual period, the ovary produces progesterone as well

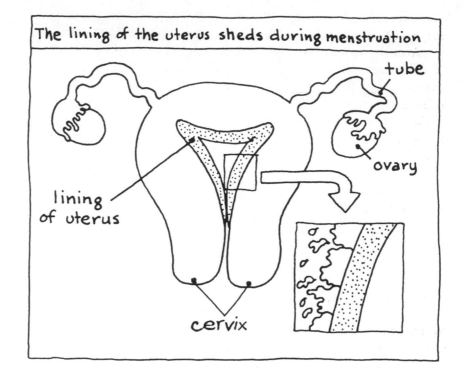

The lining of the uterus sheds during menstruation

tube

ovary

lining of uterus

cervix

as estrogen. This causes the uterine lining to prepare for pregnancy by secreting special fluids and stabilizing the growth of the lining cells. When pregnancy does not occur, the ovaries stop their hormone production; estrogen and progesterone levels decrease rapidly, and the uterine lining loses its hormonal support and begins to break down. This lining is shed during the menstrual period, so the body can make a new nest for next month's egg cell. This is the monthly rhythm of women in their fertile years.

As women reach their mid-40s, on the average, ovulation becomes less regular, and hormonal output may vary. Many women notice their periods are closer together at this time, occurring every 21 to 25 days instead of every 28 days. The amount of bleeding may be lighter than before, but occasionally it is very heavy. Sometimes, when ovulation does not occur, a period is skipped. Failure to ovulate can also cause prolonged "spotting" and erratic bleeding, since the ovaries do not secrete progesterone until ovulation occurs. In the absence of progesterone, estrogen levels tend to rise and fall and the lining is shed very irregularly. After a time of such erratic bleeding ovulation may recur and normal periods are resumed.

Around the age of 50, menstrual periods will generally get further apart and lighter, and then stop entirely. Some women experience this final pause before 50, some after. Very few women still menstruate at age 55. When a woman has had a year or two without bleeding around age 50, she has completed the time known as menopause, and should sail smoothly into a new phase of middle life.

Many variations of bleeding patterns can occur as women enter the menopause. Some are normal; others may indicate problems. It's typical for periods to be closer together at first, with heavier bleeding from time to time. Timing may be unpredictable. Later on, periods become scantier in flow and further apart. Occasionally there is just spotting for a month or two. Some women cease menstruating abruptly, after a psychological shock or after stopping the birth control pill in their 40s.

The bleeding pattern most troublesome to women and worrisome to doctors is repeated very heavy bleeding, especially if it is irregular. This can cause discomfort and anemia, and may be the result of hormonal imbalance, uterine fibroids, or cancer. Let us consider these factors and their treatment one by one.

Hormonal Imbalance and Irregular Ovulation May Cause Heavy Bleeding

By far the most common cause of irregular heavy bleeding among women in their late 40s is lack of ovulation and a resultant hormonal imbalance. When this situation occurs the cause is usually the production of too much estrogen and too little progesterone. There are various reasons for the problem, including the natural process of aging. However, frequently factors such as excessive stress can make the situation worse. Let's examine how this problem is usually treated, and then look at how it can be prevented from recurring.

When bleeding is prolonged or very heavy in the menopausal years, most doctors will first advise a minor operation known as a dilatation and curettage (D&C) to stop the bleeding and rule out cancer. In this procedure the lining of the uterus is removed, by suction or a scraping technique, and then analyzed for any abnormality. The procedure can be done in a medical office, with local anesthesia, or in an operating room where the patient can be put to sleep. Usually cancer is not found, and everyone is greatly relieved. However, after a D&C the uterine lining will grow back, and irregular bleeding may recur.

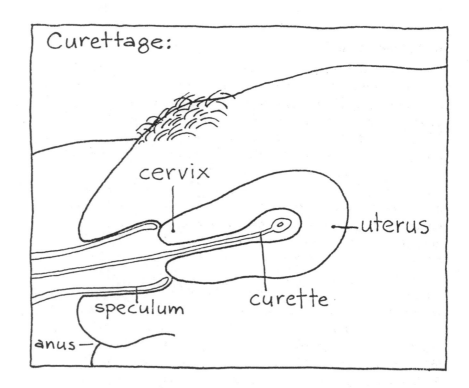

At this point the woman is often advised to take a hormone supplement called a progestin — similar to progesterone. Since progesterone, secreted by the ovary after ovulation, stabilizes the growth of the uterine lining, the use of a progestin usually stops irregular bleeding. The body responds as if ovulation had occurred. The progestin is taken for one or two weeks and when it is stopped, bleeding will recur, usually lasting less than a week, like a normal period. In many cases the irregular bleeding will not return in the next cycle. If it does, the progestin can be taken again. Occasionally the use of progestin may cause feelings of fatigue, increased appetite, and other symptoms, but there are seldom serious side effects.

Since many women would prefer to prevent such problems rather than take medicines when they occur, let's examine some natural remedies that make hormone imbalance and abnormal bleeding less likely.

Reduce emotional upsets

Emotional upset can have a profound effect on the reproductive system, causing little or no bleeding in some women and excessive or prolonged bleeding in others. Why is this so? In our long evolutionary history it has been better for the human species that fewer pregnancies occur in times of great social or personal disruption, or during prolonged episodes of exertion, exhaustion, famine, or fear. These protective mechanisms are still at work in our bodies. When we experience strong and prolonged negative emotions, the area in the brain that controls ovarian function may not operate well; ovulation may become irregular, and various hormonal problems can occur. Menstrual periods may stop completely or bleeding may be erratic and persistent. When the stressful situation is resolved, women often resume a more regular bleeding schedule. For older women, this will mean a smoother transition into the menopause.

How do you resolve the stress of a serious family illness, an angry marriage, or overwhelming financial problems? Each of us must find our own way, giving ourselves time to consult our inner wisdom. Sometimes counseling is an answer, sometimes prayer or meditation, sometimes decisive action. When a start toward resolution is made, many disturbed body functions will improve.

Quit smoking

Smokers often have problems with abnormal bleeding. Substances in cigarette smoke, such as nicotine and carbon monoxide, enter the blood stream and are damaging to the ovaries, causing them to stop ovulating too early. Hence smokers enter the menopause earlier than non-smokers and may have a more difficult time. Cigarette smoking also affects the adrenal glands and the central nervous system, causing tension, rapid pulse, and easy exhaustion. All these factors make women more susceptible to irregular bleeding.

If you drink, be very moderate

Drinking alcohol in small amounts on social occasions is a pleasure for many people. However, alcohol in large quantities has a toxic effect on many body systems. It affects the ovaries, causing a decline in ovulation and hormone production. As a consequence, heavy drinkers often experience irregular and erratic bleeding, which usually clears up when the drinking stops.

As we age we are more affected by drugs of all kinds, including alcohol, because our bodies break them down and excrete them more slowly. In the menopause it's wise to drink only small amounts (a little wine or beer on social occasions) and to quit entirely if you have bleeding problems.

Claire began to have extremely heavy and irregular periods at age 48. She worked as a waitress so she needed a lot of energy every day, but during her periods she felt exhausted. A discussion and physical exam revealed that she was very worried about money and was drinking too much. Her husband was out of work and they both drank beer all evening. They ate frozen dinners or cheese and crackers—whatever was easiest. Claire listened dubiously as I explained that alcohol, stress, and poor nutrition might be affecting her menstrual cycles. She tried taking progestins but the problem came back whenever she stopped. Finally her husband got a new job and decided to join AA. Claire went to some meetings with him and also decided to quit drinking. They both began to eat a healthier diet. In about three months Claire's periods were back to normal, and subsequently she started the menopause without further problems.

Cut down on caffeine

We know a lot about the effects of caffeine (in coffee, tea, some cola drinks, and chocolate) on the nervous system, the heart, and the digestive system. It stimulates the brain to think more rapidly, banishes fatigue, and causes muscle tension. It stimulates the heart to beat more rapidly and forcefully, sometimes causing unpleasant feelings of pounding and skipped beats. It causes more acid secretion in the stomach, worsening the problem of ulcers.

But what does caffeine do to the woman's reproductive system? There is very little research in this area, except for recent suggestions that large amounts of coffee in pregnancy may cause birth defects. Many doctors believe excessive caffeine intake in mid-life may cause constant feelings of tension and hyper-sensitivity to stimuli; this chronic stress can lead to disturbances in the output of hormones and to menstrual irregularities. Some women find that irregular heavy menstrual bleeding reverts to normal when they stop overstimulating their nervous systems with caffeine. Frequently people who drink a lot of coffee or tea also smoke cigarettes and then use alcohol to calm their "coffee nerves." The woman with bleeding problems needs to become free of dependence on all these drugs to establish a more normal menstrual rhythm or a smoother transition into the menopause.

Uterine Fibroids May Cause Heavy Bleeding

Some women in their fertile years develop irregular enlargements of the uterine muscle known as fibroids (also called myomas, or fibromyomas). Fibroids are almost never cancerous. Their growth is stimulated by ovarian hormones, especially estrogen. As a result, their growth generally diminishes in the late forties, as estrogen levels drop, and they actually shrink after the menopause, rarely creating any further problems.

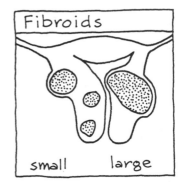

Some women who do not have distressing symptoms with fibroids are advised by their doctors to have the uterus removed, simply because it is enlarged or "it is no longer a useful organ after childbearing is over." In such situations it is a good idea to seek a second opinion from another doctor, and to remember that the uterus will shrink significantly in size after the menopause. Often it is possible to avoid surgery by simply waiting.

Some fibroids, however, enlarge to the size of a five-month pregnancy or more, which can cause significant abdominal swelling and may place uncomfortable pressure on the bladder or bowel. Fibroids can also cause very heavy menstrual bleeding, which may result in severe anemia or make it difficult for a woman to carry on her daily activities. Profuse bleeding is often the result of so-called submucous fibroids, which lie just below the uterine lining and distort the normal shape of the uterine cavity. Any woman with very heavy periods should take supplemental iron, and have her doctor check her blood count at regular intervals. Sometimes medicines such as a progestin or danazol will help to check heavy bleeding. However, if the bleeding or other symptoms from fibroids are severe, the woman may opt for some kind of surgery. A variety of surgical treatments are currently available.

If the woman wants to retain her uterus and her fertility, she can choose a myomectomy, a surgical operation in which the fibroids are removed but the uterus remains. This operation requires considerable technical skill on the part of the gynecologist, since it is important that all fibroids be removed, including very small ones that may be hard to detect. On rare occasions the operation becomes so technically difficult that the gynecologist is forced to do a hysterectomy after all, removing the entire uterus. After a myomectomy (or a hysterectomy) there is a four-to-six-week recovery period before the woman has regained all her former strength. And there is a chance that the fibroids may grow back in future years, although this risk diminishes as the woman approaches her menopause. If menstrual bleeding was very heavy before a myomectomy, this situation is often improved after the operation. If the woman becomes pregnant, she may need to have a cesarean section for the delivery of the baby if the uterus has been significantly weakened by the myomectomy surgery. Myomectomy operations have become much more popular in recent years, as more women are waiting until 35 or 40 to have children, or are opting to retain their reproductive organs even if they don't want children.

Women with very heavy menstrual bleeding who want the most minimum surgery have another option, a new technique utilizing a surgical laser. The laser beam destroys the uterine lining, removing most of it on a permanent basis so that little or no menstrual bleeding returns. The woman can no longer have children after this procedure. However, the rest of the uterus remains intact, and the recovery period after this surgery is much quicker — the patient leaves the hospital within one day. A similar result is obtained with the use of an instrument called a resectoscope, which cuts away the uterine lining but leaves the rest of the uterus intact. Not all gynecologists have been trained in using these new techniques — women who are interested should ask their doctor about this or call the nearest large medical center or medical school for a referral.

Some women with fibroids are happy to have their uterus removed. Heavy and painful menstrual periods, fatigue and weakness from the resultant anemia, or pelvic pain from other complications such as past uterine infections or endometriosis can make hysterectomy a welcome option. Women who are seriously considering hysterectomy should take several steps in advance whenever possible. One is to discuss with their doctor the question of retaining their ovaries if the ovaries seem normal at the time of surgery. This allows for the continued production of ovarian hormones — estrogen, progesterone, and androgens in the premenopausal years — and thus a smoother transition into menopause when that time comes. Even after menopause the ovaries continue to secrete androgenic hormones; the importance of these hormones throughout life is discussed in the next chapter.

Another question to discuss with your doctor is banking your own blood in advance, so that it can be used if you need a transfusion. If you are not anemic you can bank several units of blood in the month before your operation, thereby insuring that you will not contact any virally transmitted diseases that are occasionally hard to detect in donated blood, such as hepatitis or AIDS. The blood supply in the United States is currently well screened, so that the risk of contracting such diseases through a transfusion is very low. However, many people are deciding to bank their own blood in advance of elective surgery, to be absolutely safe.

The decision of whether or not to have a hysterectomy is a complex one, especially if the operation is not truly medically necessary. To clarify this point, a hysterectomy is often medically necessary for cancer, serious bleeding, overwhelming infection, severe pain, or other difficult problems. It is less necessary, or even optional, in many cases of fibroids or irregular bleeding that respond well to progestins. Women facing a hysterectomy should discuss this fully with their doctors; all their questions should be answered. They should also be aware that there are emotional implications in surgery of any kind, some negative and some positive. Many fear the idea of losing a part of their body, entering a hospital with its relative impersonality, and experiencing pain, weakness, and possible complications from surgery. Others see drama in the hospital atmosphere and enjoy the special attention and the mind-altering drugs they receive. Some people who dread an operation in advance feel greatly helped by it in the long run, while others feel angry or assaulted by their surgical experience. Much of this depends on the skill and caring of the doctors and nurses who attend them, and the outcome of the surgery on their health. As there are many unpredictables in this situation, it is best to have it well thought through in advance.

Overgrowth or Cancer of the Uterine Lining May Cause Heavy Bleeding

Unusually heavy, irregular, or persistent bleeding before the menopause, or bleeding that occurs unexpectedly after periods have stopped for six months or more, may be due to overgrowth or cancer of the lining of the uterus. If blood loss is excessive or if cancer is suspected, doctors recommend a D&C to identify problems like polyps (usually benign, pod-shaped growths of the uterine lining) or hyperplasia, varying degrees of abnormality of the lining. Hyperplasia is not cancer, but a condition of overactivity of the lining cells. Occasionally cancer of the uterine lining is found, and surgical removal of the uterus (hysterectomy) is recommended, along with other treatments.

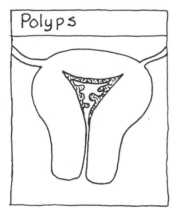

However, much of the time the diagnosis is some stage of hyperplasia, which can usually be treated with a progestin, a medicine similar to progesterone. Progestins inhibit overgrowth of the uterine lining and restore a normal pattern to the cells when taken for 10 to 14 days each month. If your doctor has suggested a hysterectomy for a non-cancerous condition such as hyperplasia, you can ask for a few courses of progestin, followed by another D&C to assess the results. Sometimes the condition clears up very easily this way.

Cancer of the Cervix May Cause Heavy Bleeding

Sometimes irregular bleeding is caused by cancer of the cervix — the lower part of the uterus at the top of the vagina (see picture on page 8). This problem is easily diagnosed by a Pap smear taken during a pelvic exam, which should be continued regularly during the menopausal years. Cervical cancer is preceded for several years by a condition known as dysplasia of the cervix, also identified by Pap smears. Dysplasia of the cervix is not cancer, but a precancerous condition of increased cellular activity, which sometimes becomes cancerous and sometimes returns to the original normal condition. Dysplasia almost never occurs in women who have never had intercourse, and is rare in women who always use a condom or diaphragm during sex, since the abnormality of dysplasia and cervical cancer is initiated by a factor that comes from a male sexual partner. This factor is suspected to be certain strains of the sexually transmitted papilloma virus, which causes genital warts in men and women.

Women with dysplasia or cancer of the cervix should obtain prompt medical treatment, which may include further diagnostic tests, freezing or laser treatment of the cervix, removal of all genital warts, removal of part of the cervix in a "cone biopsy," or hysterectomy. If a hysterectomy is not required, shielding the cervix with a condom or diaphragm in every act of intercourse will minimize further exposure to the initiating factor. If the woman is a smoker, giving up smoking will also reduce the risk, since several studies have shown a relationship between cigarette smoking and cervical cancer.

We have seen that bleeding problems in the menopause are variable and affected by many factors. Some women have virtually no bleeding problems and others have erratic episodes of spotting or flooding or both. Since some bleeding difficulties are caused by serious problems such as uterine cancer, it is wise to consult with your doctor regularly. On the other hand, it is encouraging to remember that the vast majority of bleeding problems in the menopause are the result of irregular ovulation and will be self-limited. The best method of prevention is paying attention to healthy living from day to day, as discussed in the second half of this book.

Some Positive Aspects of the Menopause, or, "The End of the Curse Is a Blessing"

The menopause is not always a problem; let's remember the positive aspects of this transition. After the menopause there are no more menstrual cramps, bleeding problems, or tampons and pads. There are no more aching pelvic discomforts with and after ovulation, no more tender breasts before a period, and no more mood swings with premenstrual tension. There are no more problems with endometriosis, fibroid tumors, birth control devices, or unwanted pregnancy. Migraine headaches tend to disappear. Not all women experience all these aggravations, but most have had some of them. Freedom from these difficulties is an aspect of the menopause to be enjoyed.

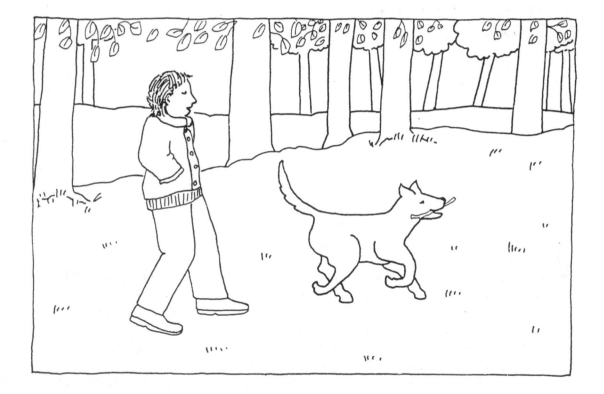

3

Janet, a 45-year-old nurse, wanted a hysterectomy because of very large fibroid tumors that were causing pressure on her bladder. Her doctor said he would also remove both ovaries as a precautionary measure against ovarian cancer later on. "You're almost in the menopause," he said, "so your ovaries won't be useful that much longer anyway." "Wait a minute," answered Janet, "I've always really liked what my ovaries have done for me. If they look normal, I want you to leave them in." Janet felt good about her decision, as she had read quite a lot about the low risk of cancer of the ovaries and the importance of these organs for general health and well being. Her doctor found her ovaries were normal and did not remove them. Janet had a smooth recovery from her hysterectomy without needing to take any replacement hormones.

*T*hroughout our lives our ovaries produce various hormones — estrogen, progesterone, and androgens — which influence general health, bone strength, sexuality, and reproduction. The ovaries also produce a tiny egg cell each month during the menstrual years, which can develop into a baby when fertilized by a sperm.

As a woman approaches the menopause these egg cells are produced less regularly. This causes changes in the timing and amount of her menstrual flow, as we discussed in the previous chapter. Finally, around age 50, no further egg cells are released. The woman's ability to bear children has ended.

At the menopause, when the ovaries are no longer producing egg cells, the secretion of estrogen and progesterone decreases greatly. However, the ovaries still play an important role at this time, because they continue to produce androgens, which influence general health and sexuality. Recent research indicates that

The Ovaries — Hidden Sources of Well-Being

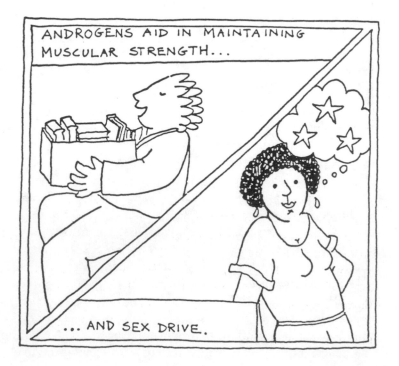

androgens are secreted in small amounts even by women in their 80s. These hormones are similar to male hormones, but definitely belong in a woman's body. They aid in maintaining muscular strength, sex drive, and the elasticity of the vagina. Androgens are also secreted by the adrenal glands located above the kidneys. This adrenal output of androgens ensures that even women without ovaries produce some of these beneficial hormones.

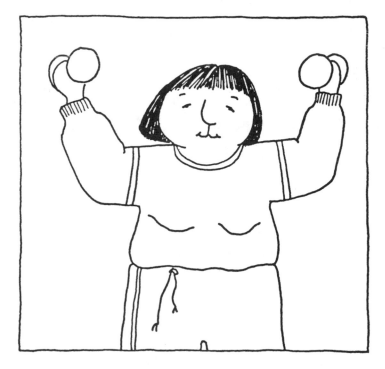

Some androgens are converted to estrogen in the body's fat cells, so women with more fat on their bodies produce more estrogen after the menopause, and may have fewer problems with hot flashes, vaginal dryness, and brittle bones. Here at last is an advantage to being fat!

But, as usual, the middle way is best. Being too fat has discomforts and hazards, including the risk of producing too much estrogen, which can cause cancer of the uterus (see Chapter 10). The best post-menopausal body is probably one that is a little plump, but still active.

In the past many doctors felt they should routinely remove the ovaries of a woman over 40 if they had to remove her uterus. They reasoned that in the menopause and beyond, the ovaries were useless organs which might become cancerous. The chance of a woman contracting cancer of the ovary in her lifetime is about one percent (it's lower in women who have borne children or taken the oral contraceptive pill, higher where there's a strong family history of ovarian cancer). Cancer of the ovary is hard to detect early and difficult to cure. Doctors reasoned that since they could give women estrogen pills to replace the hormones secreted by the ovaries, women would be better off without these organs.

New findings about post-menopausal ovaries are causing many doctors to change their views on the routine removal of healthy ovaries along with the uterus. The various hormones secreted by the ovaries in middle and old age contribute to well-being in many ways, and *cannot* always be duplicated by pills. For example, after ovarian removal some women find estrogen pills do not restore their sex drive or their strength and well-being. What they are probably missing are the ovarian androgens, for these are the hormones most connected with sexual interest and response in both sexes. Several interesting studies on androgen replacement by injection (monthly) or implant under the skin (renewed twice yearly) have been carried out by Canadian and English gynecologists. After ovarian removal, women who take androgenic hormones together with estrogen report increased energy and sexual interest compared to those taking only estrogen. However, similar studies or use of these hormones in the United States is very rare. If given orally, androgenic hormones are toxic to the liver, and their use by injection must be carefully monitored in order not to produce masculinizing side effects such as hair growth on the face, a lowered voice, or an enlarged clitoris. Some United States gynecologists prescribe 1% testosterone cream to be applied sparingly every other day to the vaginal opening, which will usually increase sex drive without other side effects.

The argument for retaining the ovaries whenever possible should be balanced by the statement that in some cases the ovaries must be removed in surgery. For example, if they do contain cancer, very large benign cysts, infection, or if they are a source of chronic pain, their removal may enhance a woman's health and chances for survival. Any patient facing a hysterectomy should discuss this question carefully with her doctor.

However, this discussion may not be easy. Many gynecologists still believe in the routine removal of ovaries after the age of 45 or 50, and some frighten their patients by saying they may get ovarian cancer if the ovaries are retained. Women faced with this dilemma should look carefully at their own situation, and ask a lot of questions. Unless there is a family history of frequent ovarian cancer, the chance of getting this disease is about one percent. If the ovaries are not diseased they will continue secreting androgens for the rest of a woman's life, which will help her bones, muscles, sexual drive, and general well-being. If her gynecologist will not listen carefully to a woman's concerns in this matter, she may need to seek a second or third opinion. While it is difficult to be at odds with your doctor, your wishes for your own body need to be respected.

The Menopause with Ovaries But No Uterus

A woman who has had her uterus removed in her 30s or 40s, but still has her ovaries, may wonder how she will know when her "change of life" is occurring. When should she expect hot flashes? What if she never gets hot flashes? How will she know when to apply the principles discussed in this book, such as taking extra calcium, exercising, or considering hormone replacement?

Generally a woman with ovaries but no uterus goes through the menopausal transition like other women. She has no more periods but her ovaries continue to function like other women's until her late 40s. At that time, when she ceases to ovulate regularly and produces less estrogen, she becomes aware of hot flashes, night sweats, and decreased vaginal secretions. If she has few symptoms of this kind (about 20% of women never get hot flashes) she can be fairly sure she has passed through the menopausal change somewhere between age 48 and 53.

Hormone therapy can be considered when symptoms occur or at age 50, whichever comes first. But no one should wait until a specific age to start exercising or eating foods high in calcium (see Chapter 7). Exercise is a good idea every day at every age. Calcium-rich foods are important for women throughout life, and calcium supplements can be started at 35 and then doubled at age 50 (see Chapter 16).

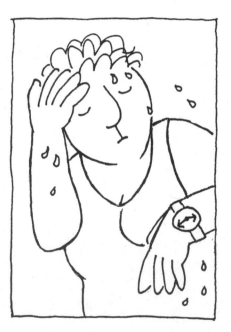

*H*ot flashes are something like adolescent acne — an outward sign of a natural process of hormonal change that all women go through as they age. We need to accept ourselves and each other in this phase of life, with open discussions and a sense of humor.

Women become more sensitive to temperature around the time of the menopause. They often feel both cold and heat more acutely, and find they are frequently adding or removing sweaters. As menstrual periods cease, about 80% of women begin to experience hot flashes — feelings of extreme heat that come on unexpectedly. During a hot flash, the face, upper body, or entire body becomes very warm and flushed. Usually this feeling lasts for two or three minutes, but it can last longer; flashes continuing for an hour have been reported by some women. Sweating will also occur — sometimes a little and sometimes a lot. Before a flash begins, a woman often feels it coming; she may need to take off her coat or sweater and fan herself — which is understandable, since her skin temperature suddenly rises 7 or 8 degrees Fahrenheit. However, the temperature inside the body does not rise, and no fever occurs. Shortly after a hot flash the body temperature actually falls a little, as explained on page 29.

All about Hot Flashes and How to Live with Them

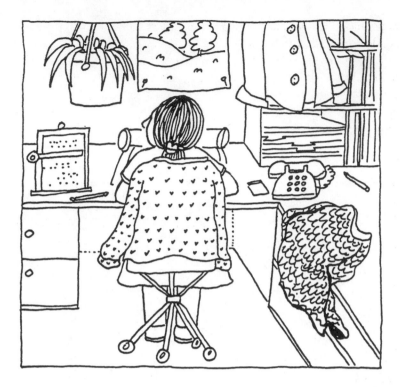

When hot flashes come at night, a woman may wake with feelings of breathlessness and heat. She often throws off her covers for a short time, and may sweat a small or large amount. Waking with frequent flashes may interrupt her sleep, which may in turn produce fatigue and difficulty concentrating during the day. Fortunately, these severe symptoms do not last long with most women, and sounder sleep is usually restored after 6 to 12 months.

In general, hot flashes are most intense and frequent in the first 2 years of the menopause, and then decrease in number and strength as the body gradually adapts to lower hormone levels and finds a new equilibrium. However, one-third of women still experience some feelings of heat as long as 9 years after the menopause.

Hot flashes need to be demystified. While they can be uncomfortable if a woman is overdressed and cannot shed some clothing, they need not be accompanied by feelings of embarrassment, anxiety, or helplessness. The popular image of the middle-aged woman as an emotional wreck, drenched in sweat and unable to cope, has been played up by pharmaceutical companies to persuade doctors and their patients to use drugs for this condition. For the younger woman this inaccurate image creates fear and dread of hot flashes. For the menopausal woman the most distressing aspect of a hot flash often is her visibility during the episode — her fear that others are noticing her and making fun of or condemning her for growing older.

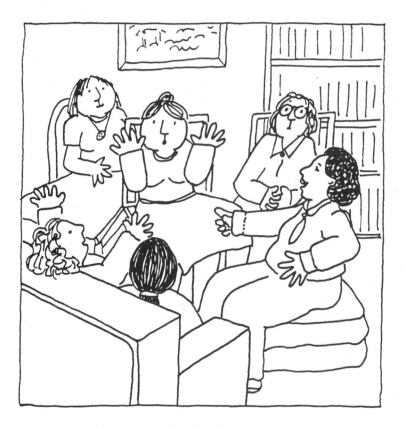

The group was talking about hot flashes. Marie said that her appearance was very important in her job as a designer, and her hot flashes had made her very self-conscious. She was greatly relieved when her doctor prescribed estrogen pills and the hot flashes went away. Sarah said that she had decided to live with the hot flash situation and had brought a small fan to work so she could turn it on whenever necessary. Several younger women in her office had asked about it and appreciated her explanation of hot flashes. Susan said that she had had three intense hot flashes during the group discussion and she wondered how bad she had looked. There was a brief silence; no one had even noticed.

Some women enjoy their hot flashes, feeling the heat as energy traveling through the body. When I have asked large groups of menopausal women about their reactions to hot flashes there are usually 2% to 3% in the audience who have a positive response! This potential for individual variability makes it important for each person to be a student of her own responses, and not to automatically expect a negative experience just because others might.

What Causes Hot Flashes?

Hot flashes begin at a time in life when there is a relatively sudden decrease in estrogen output from the ovaries. The more gradual the decrease, the less severe the symptoms. Some women with liberal amounts of body fat have fewer problems with hot flashes,

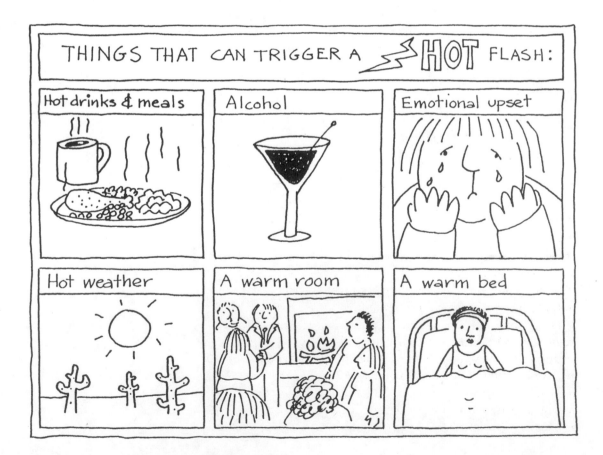

All about Hot Flashes and How to Live with Them

because their fat tissues manufacture more estrogens. On the other hand, very thin women or women who have had their ovaries removed surgically may have more problems with hot flashes. Smokers may also have more difficulty with hot flashes, because smoking reduces hormone output from the ovaries.

Although it is difficult to control or prevent hot flashes, women usually come to recognize precipitating factors. Hot drinks (especially coffee and tea), hot meals, alcohol, emotional upset, hot weather, a warm room, or a warm bed all can be triggers. Studies on the timing of hot flashes show them to be much more common between six and nine at night. Few flashes occur in the mornings on cool days, but many more occur in hot weather. All the precipitating factors mentioned here are directly or indirectly related to body temperature. Caffeine and food both raise metabolism and thereby warm the body. Alcohol causes skin flushing and makes us feel warmer. Emotional upset may do the same. Body temperature rises as the day goes on and is often at a peak in the early evening. A warm environment can also raise body temperature slightly.

What's Behind Hot Flashes?

The human body has several mechanisms to keep its internal temperature stable at an average 98.6 degrees Fahrenheit. When the outside temperature is cold, we shiver and become pale. Shivering creates heat by contracting our muscles, and a pale skin signifies that the body is keeping our blood warmer by diverting its flow to deeper tissues, thus preventing its exposure to the cold world outside. When the outside temperature is warm, we sweat and flush, cooling ourselves as sweat evaporates and blood in the skin surface loses heat to the outside. Most people barely notice these mechanisms unless the temperature is extremely cold or hot. Menopausal women, however, flush and sweat in response to heat in an exaggerated way. Their core body temperature actually falls slightly after a flash, as might be expected, thus creating a need to put on a sweater shortly after taking it off!

Why do hot flashes occur in the menopause and beyond? Has the woman's internal thermostat changed in some way? Is this response related to a "hormonal imbalance" or "deficiency state," as many have alleged? Might it have some benefits, such as

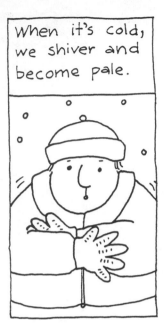

When it's cold, we shiver and become pale.

enabling older women to withstand the cold better? We do not know.

What we do know is that there is an area in the brain that regulates body temperature, keeping it in the range of 97 to 99 degrees Fahrenheit despite wide shifts in outside temperatures. This "thermostat" in the brain is adjacent to the area that governs the output of hormones by the pituitary and ovary. During the menopausal years the hormonal center may influence and throw the "thermostat" off balance, setting it lower and thus causing flashes and sweats to cool the body.

However, the story is more complex than this. Women who enter the menopause in their teens or early twenties, because of genetic reasons or surgical removal of the ovaries, rarely have hot flashes. Hot flashes occur in these women only if they take supplementary estrogen for a time and then stop taking it. The trigger for hot flashes seems to be rapid withdrawal of estrogen from a body that has grown accustomed to it. After a number of years this withdrawal effect is lessened and hot flashes become less frequent and intense.

Research into the brain mechanisms related to hot flashes has also shown that they are stimulated by a neurotransmitter known as norepinephrine, which influences the temperature-regulating center in the brain. Perhaps this helps to explain why caffeine — a drug which stimulates norepinephrine release in the body — triggers hot flashes, and why stress-reduction practices — which result in lower levels of norepinephrine — help some women reduce their hot flashes.

Living with Hot Flashes

What does this tell us about living more easily with hot flashes? Since flashes accompany a rapid decrease in estrogen, avoiding lifestyle factors that contribute to this problem will help. Smoking and excess alcohol use interfere with ovarian function. Heavy use of marijuana and some other drugs may also affect hormonal output from the ovaries. Conversely, leading a healthy and drug-free life will permit the body to adjust more gradually to the menopausal process. The daily practice of a stress reducer such as meditation or yoga is also helpful.

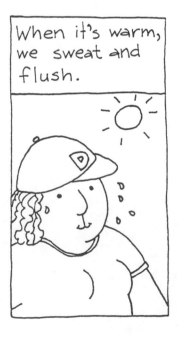

When it's warm, we sweat and flush.

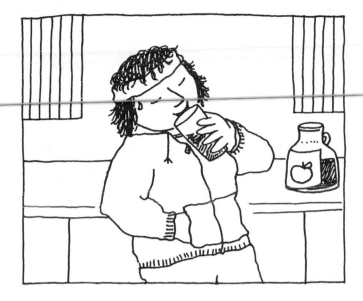

In addition, menopausal women should not be underweight. As explained in Chapter 3, estrogen is actually manufactured in body fat from other hormones after the menopause. A very thin woman will have less natural estrogen in her system, which may give her more problems with hot flashes.

Keeping cool is important for menopausal women, since all the precipitating factors in hot flashes are related to heat. Large meals, caffeine, alcohol, and strong emotions all make us warm. A menopausal woman reacts to heat by flushing and sweating in an exaggerated manner, so the most rational therapy for hot flashes is keeping cool. Don't overdress, keep the house cool, eat frequent small meals, and go easy on caffeine and alcohol. Take a cool drink of water or juice after exercise. This behavior feels good and it really helps!

Therapies for Hot Flashes

If a woman is severely troubled by hot flashes, she has several choices. She can wait for the flashes to decrease over time, which will happen naturally, or she can consider trying estrogen replacement therapy. The good news about estrogen supplements is that they will quickly decrease or eradicate hot flashes in most women. The bad news is that hot flashes return whenever the drug is stopped. However, this return may be minimized if a woman tapers off her dose of estrogen very slowly, over a period of months. The decision of whether or not to take estrogens, with its various benefits and risks, is thoroughly discussed in subsequent chapters of this book.

Some doctors prescribe medicines other than estrogen for hot flashes. A progestin can be taken, such as Norlutin (Parke-Davis) or Provera (Upjohn). These hormones also decrease hot flashes but not quite as effectively as estrogen. Side effects like fatigue, weight gain, and depression can occur. A widely advertised substitute for estrogen is Bellergal (Dorsey), which is a combina-

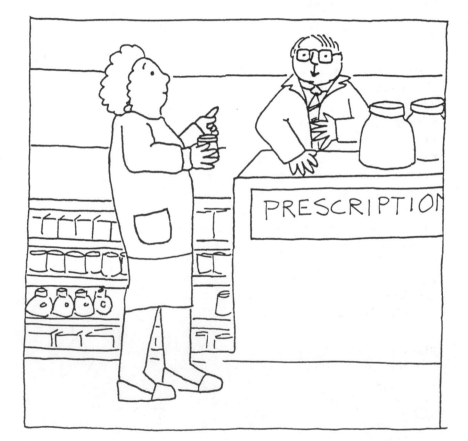

tion of phenobarbital (a habit-forming sedative), ergotamine (which contracts smooth muscle and increases blood pressure), and belladonna (which inhibits the parasympathetic branch of the nervous system, causing dry mouth, dilated pupils, constipation, and rapid pulse). Bellergal has too many side effects for continuous use, but does help some women at night if hot flashes cause severe insomnia. Clonidine (marketed as Catapres and Dixarit) is a new treatment for hot flashes, although it is primarily used for high blood pressure. Clonidine inhibits the release of norepinephrine in the brain. Side effects include sleepiness, dry mouth, and lowered blood pressure, but can be minimal in low doses. Clonidine is available as pills and in skin patches which will last for up to a week. Low doses, 0.05 to 0.15 milligrams daily, are helpful to some women with severe hot flashes who should not or do not wish to take estrogen therapy. Clonidine is a prescription drug and should be used under the guidance of a physician familiar with its side effects.

It is important to remember that all medicines that are effective have many effects on the body besides the one intended. This is also true of recreational drugs, many foods and herbal remedies. Therefore, it is important to use any medicine wisely — only when needed, in the lowest effective dose, and for the shortest time that is necessary. Consult with your doctor or nurse practitioner to find out the reasons that any medicine is prescribed for you, and its potential side effects. Use your pharmacist as a source of information as well.

Some women are interested in alternative therapies, and try various combinations of herbal medicines or vitamins for menopausal symptoms. Popular books on the menopause have suggested that Vitamin E in high doses, ginseng root, and other remedies are helpful. While there are many accounts of women who have been helped by these approaches, we do not yet have enough information on the doses and side effects involved. Like medicines, some may be helpful and others harmful. Prolonged use of high doses of ginseng, for example, has produced hypertension and other problems. All such therapies should be approached with common sense and a positive but careful attitude. Listen to the wisdom of your body, and discontinue any therapy that causes unpleasant, unbalanced feelings.

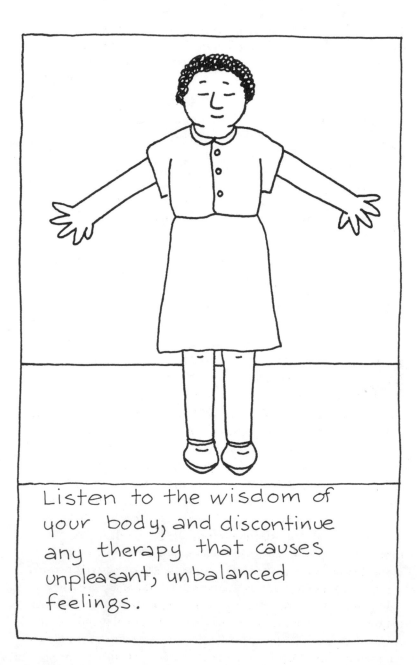

Listen to the wisdom of your body, and discontinue any therapy that causes unpleasant, unbalanced feelings.

5

The nutty thing about being an older woman as far as sex is concerned is that most women don't feel old when it comes to sex.

—Rosetta Reitz

Sex in the Second Half of Life

Will menopause mean the end of your sexuality? Not at all. Menopause is the end of a woman's fertility, or ability to become pregnant. However, she is still a sexual being capable of giving and receiving love in every way.

Sexual responsiveness changes with aging in both women and men. The sex drive may seem less urgent and arousal may take longer. However, many women continue to be sexually active into old age, both with partners and by masturbating. What is true in youth is equally true for older people — there is a tremendous individual variation in sexuality. Many women report being less interested in sex after the age of 50, feeling other aspects of their lives are more important. Others say sex is as enjoyable as ever. Some women lack a sexual partner at this time in their lives, when men their age may have sexual problems or are more difficult to find. Some turn to other women for love and companionship. Many older women masturbate for sexual pleasure.

Many women have some degree of guilt about masturbation, even in mid-life. They were probably taught in childhood that it was dirty or sinful to touch their genitals, and the resultant feelings of discomfort lingered on. Perhaps this guilt can be lessened by the realization that most people masturbate, and the practice is helpful in maintaining sexual responsiveness in mid-life. Masturbation has helped many people at times when they had no suitable sexual partners. It may even have saved a few people from unsuitable partners!

Vaginal Dryness and Lovemaking

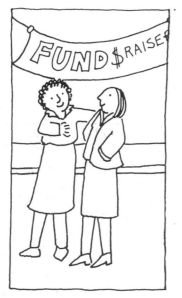

"I finally met a really good man," said Diana. "We were both taking a class at the college extension. But when we got together to make love I felt extremely sore and I had to ask him to stop. He was worried he had hurt me and I've got to do something to improve this situation. I really like him!" I examined Diana, who was 52, and found that her vaginal mucous membranes were thin and tender. I explained to her that she needed to use a small amount of estrogen cream on a regular basis, and a lubricant for intercourse. A few weeks later I bumped into Diana at a fund raiser and she was radiant. "That situation is so much better," she said. "I feel really good about myself again."

The most frequent problem women in their 50s notice during intercourse is vaginal dryness and soreness. As estrogen levels drop during the menopause and beyond, the vaginal walls become thinner and dryer. The cervix no longer secretes the quantities of mucus it did during the fertile years. The entrance to the vagina becomes smaller, especially in a woman who has not borne children. As a result, intercourse can feel painful, even though a woman is sexually responsive and can easily achieve orgasm through stimulation of the clitoral area with the hand or mouth. Lesbian women usually have less difficulty with this problem because they may not use vaginal penetration in lovemaking, or may use a small object like a finger.

Several approaches are helpful. Couples should use lubricants during foreplay and wait until the woman is thoroughly aroused before vaginal penetration. Useful lubricants are creams (unscented or scented), vegetable oils, or water-soluble jellies

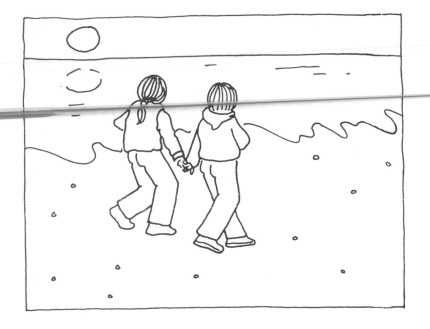

such as Lubifax or K-Y. Newer water-soluble lubricants designed specifically for sex are available through the Good Vibrations Catalog (found in the book list at the end of this book). If the couple uses the woman-on-top position, she can control the rate of insertion of the man's penis and minimize any discomfort. Many women report that regular sexual activity, either masturbation or intercourse, helps reduce vaginal soreness. If these methods are not successful, a woman should talk to her doctor about using estrogen creams (discussed in Chapter 10). These preparations are very helpful in promoting thickening of the vaginal lining, thereby reducing frictional discomfort or pain. Used in small doses under medical supervision, they can be very effective in eliminating the problem. If estrogen cannot be prescribed for some reason, a cream containing 1% or 2% testosterone is often helpful.

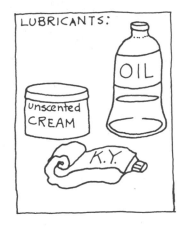

A recent study of women after the menopause revealed that those who continued to have intercourse, or to masturbate, showed fewer signs of vaginal aging than sexually inactive women. The women who continued intercourse had similar estrogen levels but higher androgen levels than those who did not. The study appears to underline two important points. First, that continuing to be sexually active through intercourse or masturbation may help to preserve vaginal function after the menopause. Second, that the ovaries — a major source of androgen secretion — remain active organs into old age.

What can couples do when their usual sexual activities become a problem? Frequently with aging the man may have more difficulties with erection, or the woman with vaginal soreness. Illness or fatigue may impair the sexual response of one or both partners. Alcohol, tranquilizers and many medications can reduce sex drive and alter men's abilities to keep an erection. These problems should be discussed with a doctor, as some people can decrease or eliminate medicines by making changes in eating and drinking habits, increasing exercise, and learning how to relax.

It is also important for couples to realize that intercourse is not the only means of sexual expression. People give affection and pleasure to each other in many other ways, and can stimulate one another with their hands, mouths, or a vibrator, and through massage with oils and creams. While the urgency to achieve

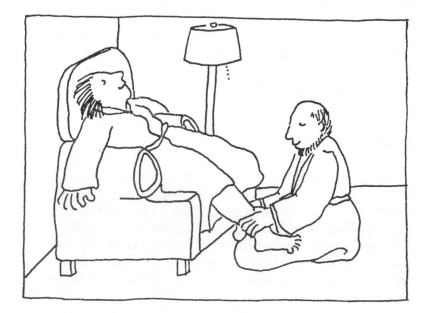

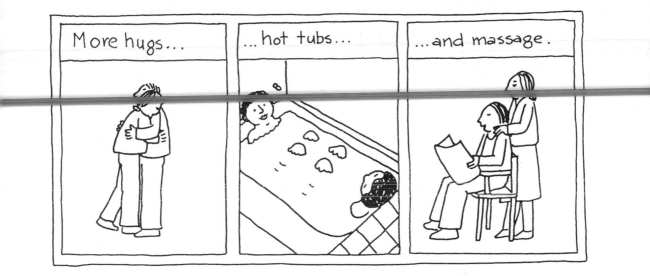

More hugs... ...hot tubs... ...and massage.

orgasm may decline with age, the gratification of giving and receiving a loving touch remains strong. Learning how to give and receive a slow, deep massage of the hand, foot, shoulders, or entire body is a wonderful experience at any age.

One of the problems with sex in younger years for many women is the lack of prolonged caressing and foreplay, and the rapidity with which sexual encounters lead to intercourse. In later life there is an opportunity to correct this imbalance. Instead of giving up on sex, couples can include more touching in their lives, more hugs, hot tubs, and massage together, and expand their definition of sensual pleasure.

Kegel's Exercises

Contracting and relaxing the muscles that surround the anus, vagina, and urethra (the opening for urine) can be very helpful. Women have found that these simple exercises increase their awareness of how to relax or to use these muscles during sex. Many have reported that it is easier to achieve orgasm after practicing Kegel's exercises. Other women say they have less tendency to develop hemorrhoids or to leak urine while coughing, laughing, or sneezing.

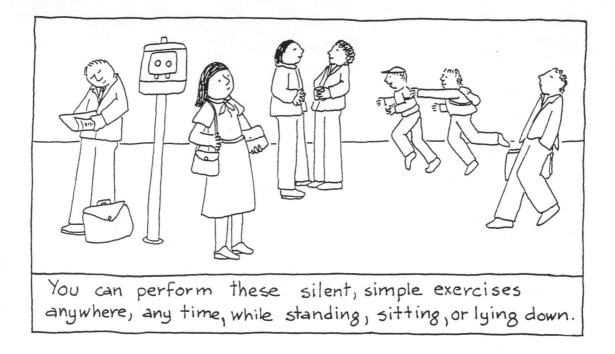

You can perform these silent, simple exercises anywhere, any time, while standing, sitting, or lying down.

Kegel's exercises, named after the gynecologist who developed them to prevent urinary incontinence, are performed as follows: imagine that you want to stop urinating, and squeeze the muscles in your vaginal area firmly. Practice this squeeze technique while counting to three — then relax. After repeating this squeeze–hold–relax technique a number of times, try a rapid alternation between tightening and letting go of the muscles. You can perform these silent, simple exercises anywhere and any time, while standing, sitting, or lying down.

Irritation, Incontinence, and Infection

Like the tissues lining the vagina, the lining of the urethra becomes thinner and less elastic after the menopause. Women may experience a need to urinate more frequently, or may have to go to the bathroom several times at night. Some have difficulty with leakage of urine when they cough, sneeze, or laugh. Urinary incontinence should be discussed with a doctor if it is severe. This can be treated with Kegel's exercises or in some cases with surgery. Estrogen or testosterone cream (see Chapter 10) may be helpful in some cases.

As the vaginal tissues become thinner and dryer after the menopause, they can easily be irritated by strong soaps. Warm (not hot) water is the best cleanser. For itching or irritated tissues, oatmeal baths are soothing (put some cooked oatmeal in a strainer and hold it under the tap as you fill the tub). Vaginal infections may occur after intercourse, especially with new partners, and often require a consultation with a doctor or nurse practitioner.

Birth Control

How long should birth control methods be used in the menopausal years? As long as menstrual periods occur and, to be on the safe side, for the next six to twelve months. However, the likelihood of becoming pregnant around age 50 is small, so couples can use simple methods such as the diaphragm, condom, or foam. An IUD, if already in place and comfortable, may be left in until periods stop, but should be removed if heavy bleeding or pain occurs. The pill should not be taken over the age of 40 in most cases, and not over 35 by smokers, because of increased risk of complications such as heart attack or stroke. Women following fertility awareness methods of birth control may have difficulty recognizing ovulation, which occurs less regularly and with lessened secretion of cervical mucus.

Hysterectomy and Sexuality

Women who are contemplating hysterectomy for other than urgent reasons should get opinions from several doctors if possible, and should know that there are some sexual side effects from hysterectomy.

While sexual pleasure leading to female orgasm is usually achieved from stimulation of the clitoris, the cervix and uterus also play a sexual role. To understand this sexual role of the uterus, we must reevaluate early theories about female response. Under the influence of Freudian theory, it was once believed that women who needed direct clitoral stimulation (as in masturbation or foreplay) to achieve orgasm were sexually immature. The "completely sexual" woman responded to intercourse alone, according to this view, which emphasized the importance of the "vaginal orgasm."

Many sexologists in recent years have pointed out that all female orgasms originate in the clitoris, which may be stimulated directly by hand or mouth, or indirectly by intercourse. Vaginal penetration is not necessary for orgasm, and by itself may not provide enough indirect clitoral stimulation for high levels of arousal. Psychologists and feminists have used these findings to counter early Freudian theories, and debunk the "myth of the vaginal orgasm." Now our views are changing again on this controversial subject! For many women there *is* something about vaginal penetration (along with clitoral stimulation) that enhances the quality of sexual pleasure and orgasm. Instead of intercourse, some women use fingers or other objects to achieve these sensations.

The extra pleasure may come not only from the physical closeness of vaginal penetration, but from the stimulation of the cervix and uterus. After a hysterectomy, this component is lost, as are the sensations from uterine contractions during orgasm. It is noteworthy that about one third of women who have had a hysterectomy report that their sexual pleasure decreased after surgery.

Women considering hysterectomy may be able to predict their own reactions in advance by self-observation. Women who find that cervical stimulation and/or deep thrusting greatly enhance the quality of their sexual pleasure may experience more loss after hysterectomy. Conversely, those for whom deep penetration and movement in intercourse is painful may have better sex after hysterectomy.

Until very recently, the uterus has been seen as primarily a reproductive organ without a sexual role. Now that we are more aware of its potential to enhance sexual experience, more research will appear to help women decide on the pros and cons of hysterectomy.

European gynecologists have given more recognition to the

sexual role played by the cervix, and frequently will perform a partial or subtotal hysterectomy when this operation is needed, removing the uterus but leaving the cervix and upper vagina intact. This operation has the added advantage of being simpler and quicker than a standard hysterectomy. However, the woman must continue to have regular Pap smears to detect cervical cancer.

If both ovaries are removed at the time of hysterectomy, a woman's sexual response is often changed. Estrogen replacement by pill or injection will relieve hot flashes and prevent vaginal soreness, but it may not entirely restore the sex drive. It is not estrogen, but androgenic hormones secreted by the ovaries and adrenal glands which make a woman feel more sexual. Androgens can be given by injection or long term implant (see Chapter 3), and this treatment is often successful in restoring sex drive. However, the dosage used must be carefully monitored as increased facial hair growth or other masculinizing symptoms can occur. Small amounts of androgen in 1% or 2% testosterone vaginal cream have often been helpful as well. (See Chapter 10.) Androgens such as testosterone should not be taken in pill form, as long term usage may prove toxic to the liver.

These findings are causing many gynecologists to reconsider the preventive removal of healthy ovaries during hysterectomy, even in menopausal women. For many years it was believed that any decrease in sex drive women felt after such surgery was psychological, and that all problems could be solved by counseling and estrogens. We are now less sure of these precepts and are coming to appreciate more the intricately connected wisdom of the body.

"I had to have it all taken out," explained Christie, "because I had a terrible infection from my IUD. But sex isn't quite the same as it used to be. I don't experience the same excitement at certain times of the month, and I miss the feeling of contractions deep inside. Still, I think I'm retraining myself to feel what I felt before." "How do you do that?" I asked. "I can't really explain it," she answered, "but I imagine what it used to feel like and try to match it." "Carry on," I said. We both laughed.

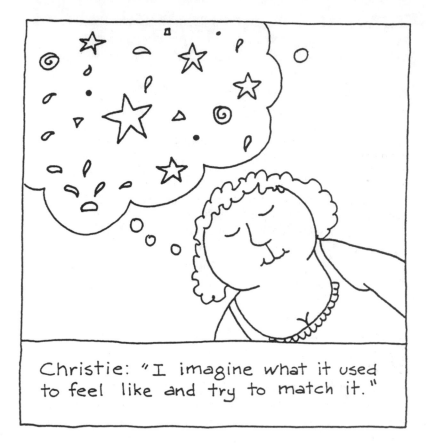

Christie: "I imagine what it used to feel like and try to match it."

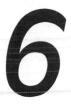

After her husband died Eileen felt neutered inside. She found she had lost interest in her appearance and in trying to relate to men. She had felt gray inside and out for several years, until she met Jonathan in a folk dance class. He wasn't perfect; she would never marry him, but he helped her to feel alive again in an important way. She bought some new clothes and went to an exercise class. Her depression lifted and life began to glow. Her friends told her she looked wonderful. This is amazing, she said to herself. It's all still there, even at 55. This realization transformed her life in a subtle, positive way.

Age Is Becoming... Your Looks in the Menopausal Years

What will menopause do to our looks? Will the hormonal changes leave us fat, wrinkled, stiff, and sexually unappealing?

Not necessarily. Women who have an early menopause due to surgical removal of the ovaries at 25, for example, still look 25 despite their hormonal loss. It is not the menopause but the aging process that most affects our appearance. Aging occurs at different rates in different people. Although genetic factors play a role in this, the crucial determinants of our appearance as we age seem to be health and happiness. We all get old and look old, but it can happen more or less beautifully, depending on our inner environment. Let's look at the questions about appearance.

Weight Gain

Weight gain can occur at the menopause but it is not necessarily inevitable. In our culture most people gain weight throughout their middle years because they exercise too little and eat too rich a diet. With aging we tend to reduce body movement more than food intake. Before blaming this on the menopause, let's examine what role the sex hormones play in body weight.

Studies done on menstruating women show they are more active physically in the first two weeks after their periods, when estrogen is the predominant hormone in their systems. After ovulation, when progesterone is also produced by the ovaries, activity slows down and food intake increases; the body is preparing itself for pregnancy. Many women find they lose a little weight after menstruation and then gain weight before their periods due to these hormonal influences. For women on the birth control pill, taking a progestin with estrogen for the whole month, weight gain is common.

But what about the menopause? At this time estrogen levels fall sharply, and progesterone almost disappears from the system. Not only do we lose the subtle influence of estrogen to stimulate physical activity, but also the progesterone effect, which causes increased appetite and a slower pace. The net effect of the two hormones was to maintain weight levels, with a slight seesaw effect. After the menopause, the seesaw effect is gone, but there is no hormonal reason for continued weight gain. We are on our own, needing to balance food intake with exercise. This doesn't necessarily mean a stringent diet for the rest of our lives. It means eating lots of the right foods (whole grains, vegetables, fruits, and skim milk products) and little as possible of the wrong foods (fats, sugars, refined flours, and rich meats). It means lots of walking, bending, and other movement. In societies where this happens naturally, many people become thinner after the menopause rather than fatter.

Women who take estrogens after the menopause have been studied for the effect of these hormones on their body weight.

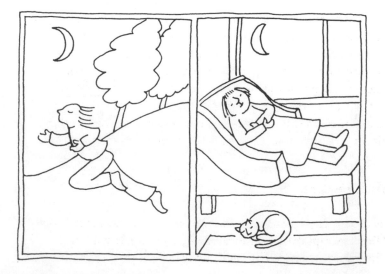

Age Is Becoming...Your Looks in the Menopausal Years

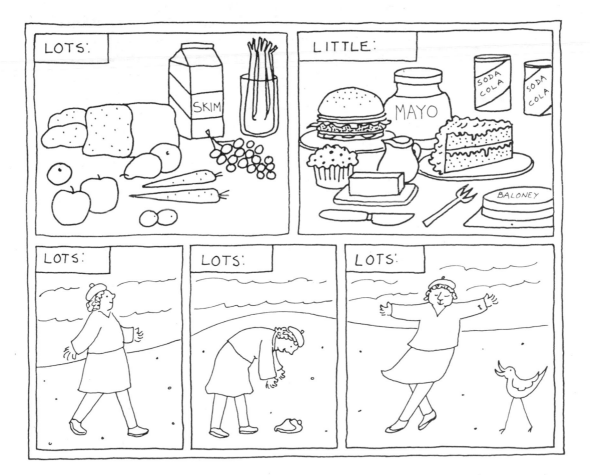

They have been found to weigh significantly less than women of a comparable age not on estrogens. However, most of these studies so far have been done on older women taking estrogens alone, without added progestin. In recent years it has become apparent that a progestin should be added to estrogen in the last 10 to 14 days of each month to minimize the cancer risk. Under these circumstances some weight gain may occur, which might minimize the differences between hormone users and non-users.

Skin Changes

Another common concern about the menopause is that the skin will become rapidly dry and wrinkled. In younger women the sex hormones produced by the ovaries have various effects on the

48

skin. Estrogen has the effect of liquefying the waxy material produced in skin cells and thereby reducing the severity of blackheads and acne. Androgens, also produced by the ovaries, make acne worse. After the menopause, when both hormones are reduced, facial pimples are rarely a severe problem. Dryness and thinning of the skin due to lessened amounts of fat beneath it often accompany aging. The menopause does play a part in this process, but the changes are gradual.

The two most common causes of wrinkling and aging of skin are smoking and excess exposure to sunlight. Smoking decreases blood supply to skin cells by constricting small blood vessels throughout the body. In addition, the blood of a smoker conveys less oxygen and more carbon monoxide than is normal. Skin cells and their underlying elastic layer are thus undernourished and lose their moisture and their natural contour, resulting in wrinkles. After the age of 30 or 35, the skin of smokers and non-smokers begins to look different. Next time you are on an airplane, notice the skin of people sitting in the non-smoking and smoking sections as you walk up and down the aisle. "Crow's feet" wrinkles around the eyes, lines and creases, and a blue-gray color due to poor oxygenation are all more apparent among smokers. The color difference can be reversed when smoking is stopped, but the wrinkles remain.

Exposure to the sun is the most significant cause of skin wrinkling. People with brown or black skin are more protected from this effect and often have a smooth, youthful skin into old age. Caucasians, with lighter skin coloring, are more prone to skin damage from sun exposure. Sunburn damages the elastic layers underneath skin cells, causing them to become less supportive of the skin itself. Fair-skinned people who work outdoors all their lives often have more wrinkled, weather-beaten skin. They also are more likely to develop skin cancer. Some sunshine is healthy and promotes vitamin D formation in the skin, but sunburn can cause problems. People with fair skin should wear hats and protective clothing or sunscreen lotions on bright days.

Finally, general health and nutrition affect our skin as we age. Virtually all essential nutrients are needed for the health of our cover layer. People who ignore the precepts of healthy eating and living but take large amounts of one or two vitamins or minerals are not helping their skin and appearance as much as people who eat a variety of whole natural foods and take a balanced vitamin/mineral supplement as needed.

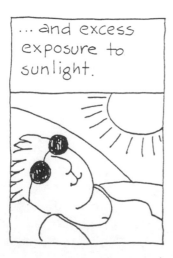

The two most common causes of wrinkling and aging of skin are smoking...

... and excess exposure to sunlight.

Many people know vitamin A plays a role in the health of skin, eyes, and mucous membranes. However, this fat-soluble vitamin can be stored in the body, and excessive amounts from animal sources or vitamin pills can be dangerous. Most people should not take more than 15,000 IU daily as a supplement. It is better to get most vitamin A from foods like carrots, sweet potatoes, yellow squash, yellow and red fruits, peppers, and all deep green, leafy vegetables.

Use of moisturizing skin cream is helpful for dry skin. Excessive hot water and soap wash away protective natural skin oils and should be avoided. Some cosmetics contain many chemicals which can be absorbed through the skin. Nothing will improve your appearance as much as a walk in the open air, healthy food, and activities that bring happiness and relaxation.

Loss of Flexibility

Changes in body flexibility — in the movement of joints and the elasticity of muscles — do occur with aging, but can be counteracted with stretching and exercise. It is not the menopause that creates stiffness and joint pain so much as our habits of living, including insufficient movement, excess weight, and the wrong foods. A gradual program of stretching, such as yoga, and daily walking can restore a flexible body.

Sex Appeal

Many women worry about losing their sex appeal after menopause. But sex appeal is a subtle force, made up of many variables, including interest in sexuality, transmitted verbally and by body language, and warmth and interest in others. These factors need not change with the menopause. There are, however, hormonal factors which act as subtle sex attractants in younger women. At the time of ovulation, when estrogen levels are high, women secrete an odor which attracts men, even though they are not aware of the smell. These sex attractants are known as pheromones; their effects can be easily seen in the animal world when a female is "in heat" and fertile. Studies with human couples have shown that men initiate intercourse more often during a woman's fertile time. This source of sexual attraction is lost after the menopause. However, the use of subtle perfumes may stimulate the same areas in the brain as the pheromones did, giving out the same message of sexual receptivity. Among humans the most important sexual organ is the mind — most of our turn-ons and turn-offs are related to our thought processes. If you are interested in sexuality, you can be sure the menopause will not create a sudden end to your sex appeal.

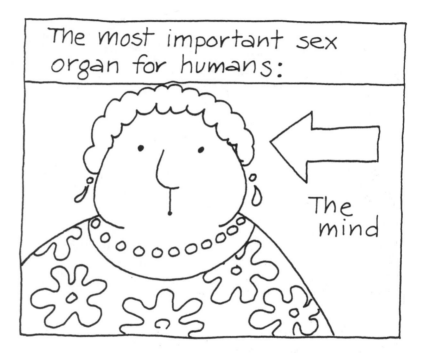

The message of this chapter is that physical appearance does change with aging, but not markedly with the menopause itself. The changes that come about with aging are minimized by healthy living and a sense of meaning in life, which is why some old people look young and — some young people look old.

7

After the menopause women are more likely to develop osteoporosis — a condition in which bones lose their strength and fracture easily. "Osteon" is the Greek word for bone, and "porosis" means full of tiny holes, or porous. Bones which have osteoporosis are more likely to break, bend, or become compressed, leading to pain and disability.

The Biology of Osteoporosis

Why do older women develop osteoporosis? Throughout life our bones are constantly being remodeled — they are not inert organs despite their apparent rigidity. At certain times calcium is dissolved out of our bones to replenish the calcium supply in the blood, and in this process bone becomes weaker. This happens when our diets are too low in calcium and when we are physically inactive. Reducing diets are often deficient in calcium and are responsible for bone loss in many women. At other times increased amounts of calcium enter the bones from the blood stream, making them denser, stronger, and larger. This happens when we do physical work and exercise, and also when there is plenty of calcium in our diets.

Keep Your Bones Strong... How to Avoid Osteoporosis

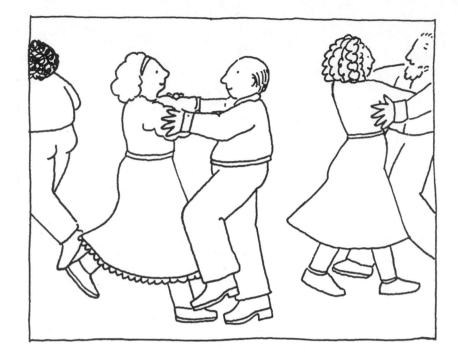

Erica was worried about developing brittle bones, or osteoporosis. Her mother had lost considerable height with aging and had back pain whenever she walked any distance. "What can I do if I don't want to take estrogen?" asked Erica. "I've heard that lots of calcium and a vegetarian diet are helpful." "You're right on that score," I said. "Another thing you can do is to exercise every day." "I haven't really exercised in years," groaned Erica. "Isn't it dangerous to start suddenly?" "Start with a walking program," I suggested, "and work up to 30 minutes a day at a brisk pace. Find something you really enjoy, like dancing or hiking, for the weekends. Start slowly and keep it up."

Calcium is a mineral with many functions. Besides giving strength to bones and teeth, it is dissolved in blood and body fluids where it plays a role in muscle contraction, the function of the heart, the transmission of nerve impulses, and the blood-clotting system. The body has many glandular systems which regulate and stabilize the calcium level in the blood, pulling it in and out of bones and in and out of our digestive tracts.

At the time of the menopause there is a steep drop in estrogen production in women. Among its many functions, estrogen plays a major role in preserving bone strength through constant calcification. When estrogen is no longer abundant, bones dissolve more rapidly than they recalcify, and a woman's bones may become softer, weaker, and more likely to break. Why does estrogen play such an important role in keeping our bones strong? No one is sure, but it is probably a mechanism to protect the bones from excessive calcium loss during pregnancy, and to create rapid recalcification of bone between the end of breast-feeding and the next pregnancy. At these times estrogen levels in the body are high. While a woman is breast-feeding, her estrogen levels are low and calcium leaves the bones to go into milk formation.

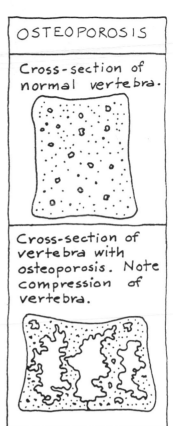

OSTEOPOROSIS

Cross-section of normal vertebra.

Cross-section of vertebra with osteoporosis. Note compression of vertebra.

After menopause, when estrogen levels drop, about 25% of white, Asian, and brown-skinned women develop serious osteoporosis. Black women rarely develop this problem, for reasons we don't entirely understand. As a race Blacks have thicker bones, which gives them a selective advantage against fractures. Susceptible women may fracture their wrists after a fall or milder trauma; this commonly occurs in the 50s. In their 60s, women may experience back pain as a result of the loss of calcium in their vertebral bones, with "crush fractures" or severe compression of these bones of the spine. Loss of height and a humped back may result. While about 20% of women show vertebral compression by age 70, severe pain or disability is rare; many women are not aware of having the condition. The most significant bone problem occurs typically after age 70 when fracture of the head of the thigh bone or femur, commonly known as fracture of the hip, may take place. Fifteen percent of white women will fracture their hip in their later years, and one-tenth of such patients will die from complications of the fracture. Those who recover are often permanently limited in their ability to walk without pain. Black and Latina women have a lower risk of hip fracture.

Osteoporosis can also cause tooth loss, which is more common in women than in men after age 50, and also more common in smokers. The weakened bone structure in the jaws of women with osteoporosis permits loosening and ultimate loss of teeth.

Clearly there are significant problems associated with osteoporosis in some older women. How can we identify the 25% of women who are at risk of incurring fractures with aging due to osteoporosis?

Who's at Risk?

Medical scientists are working on screening tests to identify those at greater risk of fractures. At this writing, there is much debate but no agreement about the utility of *any* x-ray or laboratory tests to predict who is going to have osteoporotic fractures in the future.

A variety of x-ray techniques have been developed in recent years which are designed to screen women at the time of menopause, in order to identify those who are losing bone most rapidly and may therefore be most at risk for fractures. These tests may be helpful in predicting vertebral compression fractures of the spine, but are not considered useful in predicting hip fractures. One test commonly used is called dual-photon absorptiometry or DPA, which measures the density of bone in the vertebrae of the low back. The other test is the more widely known computed tomography or CT scan, which surveys the same vertebrae using a different radiological technique. While both tests have certain advantages and disadvantages, I prefer the DPA test as it subjects the patient to significantly less radiation than the CT scan. If a woman has a bone screening test such as a DPA or CT at the onset of menopause and again a year later, the tests may help identify whether she is a rapid bone loser who could benefit from hormones, or a slow bone loser who might not need them to prevent subsequent vertebral crush fractures. However, it should be understood that these tests are subject to a certain percentage of errors, which makes it difficult for them to accurately detect small changes in bone density. At present they are not considered truly predictive for fractures — they only indicate an increased or decreased risk based on preliminary data. Many women with low bone density avoid fractures, and some with high bone density sustain them.

Because of the growing interest in osteoporosis, many new programs designed for mass screening with DPA or CT have been developed and promoted in recent years. However, since the information collected so far does not allow accurate predictions of who will have a fracture, it is not ethical to advocate that large numbers of midlife women take and pay for these tests. Bone screening tests by x-ray tend to cost over $200 and are rarely reimbursed by medical insurance companies.

Biochemical tests for prediction of rapid bone loss after menopause are also under evaluation, and promise to be less expensive than x-ray studies. Measurements of body fat, estrogen levels in the blood, and the excretion of calcium or other products in the urine, calculated in a special way, can all be helpful in determining who may be at risk. Women with more body fat tend to have higher estrogen levels and less problem with brittle bones! At present most of these tests are only beginning to be used, so their validity in predicting fracture rates is still under investigation. We will be hearing more about these tests in coming years, which will help doctors and women decide who is most at risk.

Because of the lack of tests that can validly predict fracture risk, most thoughtful doctors rely on genetic and lifestyle factors — such as race, body build, and use of alcohol or cigarettes — to help decide who is most at risk for brittle bones. The table on page 56 summarizes these factors, which will be discussed individually. Read the table with care, noting how it applies to you individually.

Genetic and medical factors

All ethnic groups except Blacks are at higher risk for osteoporosis. Black women rarely develop the problem, perhaps because of heavier bones or favorable hormonal differences. Latina women from Central America also have a lower risk of fracture.

Women who have had a previous fracture that occurred easily — from a minor fall, light blow, or twisting motion — may already have some osteoporosis.

Women with female relatives who had fractures or significant height loss with aging may inherit a family tendency toward osteoporosis. However, there is no good research so far which shows that osteoporosis runs in families.

Women who are slim, with small muscle mass, are more at risk of osteoporosis than heavier, more muscular women. This is especially true if they are short and thin, as their total body weight is less. Several reasons are obvious here — more weight means more gravitational pull on the body and more work for the bones and muscles — all of which keep the bones calcified. More fat means more estrogen production within the body which helps prevent osteoporosis (see Chapter 3). The slender smoker is at

Genetic or Medical Factors	*Life Style Factors*
Being in a non–Black ethnic group	High alcohol use
Previous fractures that occurred easily, without major trauma	Smoking
Female relatives with osteoporosis	Lack of exercise
Being thin (especially if you are short)	Low calcium diet
Early menopause (before age 40)	Lack of Vitamin D from sun, diet, or pills
Chronic diarrhea or surgical removal of part of the stomach or small intestine	Very high protein diet
Kidney disease with dialysis	High salt diet
Daily use of cortisone	Never having borne children
Daily use of thyroid (over 2 grains), Dilantin, or aluminum-containing antacids	High caffeine use (over 5 cups daily)

greatest risk, and the obese non-smoker at lowest risk of bone fractures.

Women with an earlier menopause often have more osteoporosis, since they lose bone over a longer period of time.

Patients with chronic diarrhea, such as ulcerative colitis or Crohn's disease, absorb less calcium and lose more in their stools. The same problems can occur if part of the intestinal tract has been removed by surgery. Patients on kidney dialysis can develop calcium deficiency and need special care for this problem. Patients who use cortisone daily in significant amounts develop osteoporosis. Women on high daily doses of thyroid may develop osteoporosis, although the evidence for this is incomplete. Dilantin and aluminum-containing antacids are other medicines that cause decalcification of bone.

Lifestyle factors

Let's look at lifestyle — the daily habits that cause osteoporosis, as well as those that increase bone strength.

High alcohol use contributes to osteoporosis and bone fractures. Alcohol acts directly on bone cells, suppressing the growth of new bone. Excess alcohol is toxic to the ovaries, causing infrequent ovulation and menstrual irregularities in younger women, as well as decreased breast size. The menopausal woman who uses alcohol heavily may have less hormonal output from her ovaries, and as a result will have more problems with hot flashes, vaginal soreness, and rapid loss of calcium from her bones. Many people who drink heavily do not pay attention to their diets, which compounds the problem of loss of calcium from bones. Finally, heavy use of alcohol leads to accidents, falls, and fractures. Many hip fractures in older women are caused by falls related to the use of alcohol or tranquilizers.

Smoking contributes to osteoporosis. First of all, smokers have a decreased estrogen level in their blood and tissues and an earlier menopause. Several studies have shown significantly higher rates of bone fractures in post-menopausal smokers, probably because of harmful effects of smoking on the ovaries

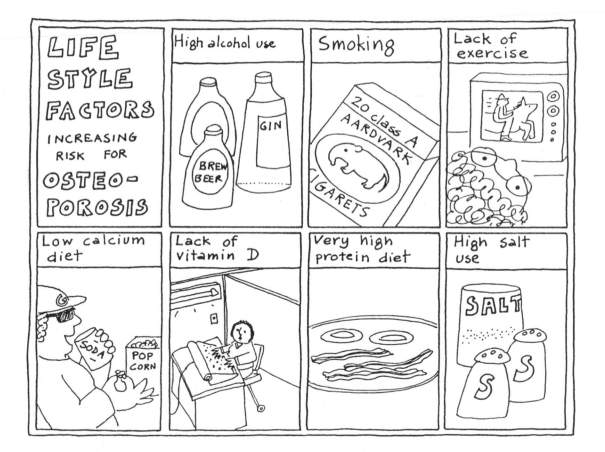

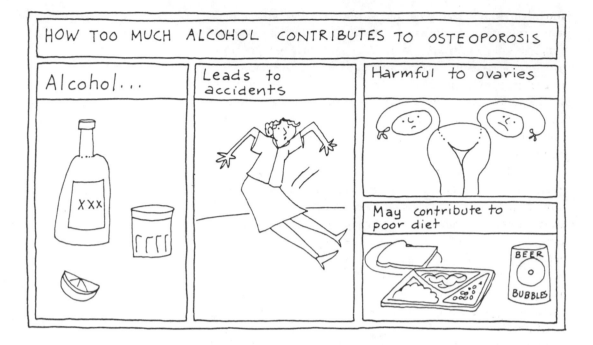

HOW TOO MUCH ALCOHOL CONTRIBUTES TO OSTEOPOROSIS

Alcohol...

Leads to accidents

Harmful to ovaries

May contribute to poor diet

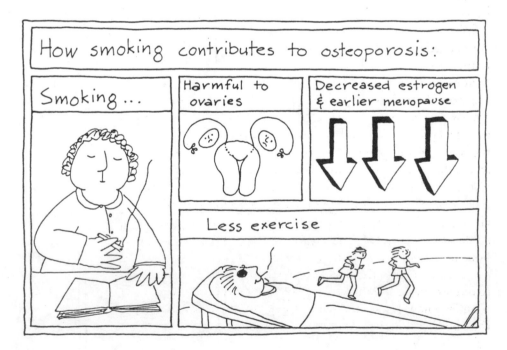

How smoking contributes to osteoporosis:

Smoking...

Harmful to ovaries

Decreased estrogen & earlier menopause

Less exercise

Keep Your Bones Strong...How to Avoid Osteoporosis

and other glands, including the parathyroid glands in the neck which regulate calcium levels in the blood. Since smokers tend to weigh less and exercise less than non-smokers, their risk of osteoporosis is higher on this account. Thin smokers are at special risk for fractures.

Lack of exercise can cause osteoporosis. When people are inactive during illness, their bones will lose calcium just as their muscles will become weaker. Conversely, when we walk, run, jump, dance, or otherwise jar our skeletons, a mild electrical energy charge develops along the bone which stimulates bone growth and calcification. This electrical energy effect is sometimes utilized by orthopedic surgeons to promote more rapid healing of fractures, by running a very low electrical current along the shaft of an injured bone. Our arms as well as our legs need exercise to keep our bones strong. Tennis players have significantly thicker bones in the arm that holds the racket. Similar effects can be achieved through energetic swimming, gardening, lifting, Nautilus, working out with weights, and other upper-body exercise. Jogging or walking while moving the hands holding small weights is also useful; this form of exercise is called "heavy hands."

A very interesting study was done at the University of Wisconsin by Dr. Everett Smith. He studied women in a nursing home, average age 80, by measuring the size and calcification of their bones with an x-ray technique. One group of women exercised their arms and legs for thirty minutes three times a week *sitting in their chairs,* a second group took extra calcium, and a control group made no changes in their diet or exercise. While the control group lost bone calcium during the three years of the study, the exercise group and the calcium group both gained bone, the exercise group most of all. When you consider that these women were about 80 years old and exercised from their chairs, the results are very encouraging. Many other recent studies also show that a consistent exercise program can increase bone mass before and after the menopause.

Clearly, part of the current problem of osteoporosis is related to our sedentary lives and our reliance on motors instead of feet. Women who leave all the "heavy work" for men are not using their bodies enough or doing the best for their bones. Exercise

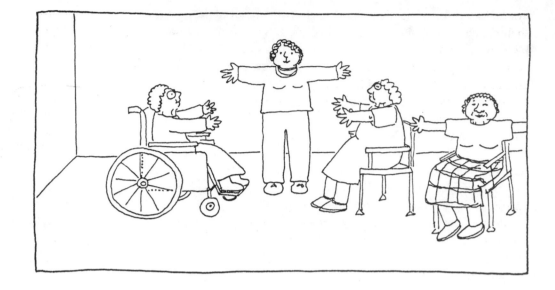

should be a lifelong commitment, planned for every day. Chapter 14 gives more suggestions on how to begin and maintain a joyous and self-perpetuating plan for movement.

A low-calcium diet can also contribute to osteoporosis. Elderly people who subsist on tea, toast, lunch meat, and canned fruit may be in short supply of this nutrient. International studies have shown that countries with a low-calcium diet, like Japan, have more problems with osteoporosis and fractures than countries with a high-calcium diet, like Finland.

Calcium is contained in many common foods which should be consumed regularly by women of all ages. If you eat plenty of foods containing calcium in your teens, twenties, and thirties, and exercise regularly, you will reach menopause with bones of maximum strength. But even if you haven't paid much attention to calcium in your diet up to now, begin at once! As the table below shows, a wide variety of foods are good calcium sources; you can get plenty of calcium from healthful and tasty foods even if you don't like milk products. Calcium-fortified orange juice is now on the market, providing as much calcium per ounce as milk. Studies indicate that this calcium is well absorbed.

Many other foods are also good sources of calcium. However, spinach, chard, beet greens, parsley, rhubarb, and chocolate are not included here since their calcium is poorly absorbed due to their oxalic acid content.

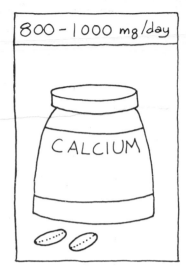

The Recommended Daily Allowance for calcium is 800 milligrams, but most nutritionists believe that women should take in 1,000 to 1,500 milligrams daily during their adult life to optimize their bone strength. Since many people cannot take in this much calcium from food alone, calcium supplements are often recommended for the woman over 35. They generally come as 500-milligram tablets, and are best absorbed if taken with food. Calcium in the form of calcium carbonate or calcium citrate is easily found in pharmacies and health food stores. Some samples of calcium from bonemeal and dolomite have contained lead and other contaminants and are not currently recommended.

Whether a high calcium diet at the time of menopause will protect against bone loss is debatable. Ideally, the high calcium

Common Foods High in Calcium

Food	Amount	Calcium Content
skim milk powder	¼ cup	400 mg
low-fat milk	1 cup	350 mg
yogurt	1 cup	300 mg
low-fat cottage cheese	1 cup	120 mg
collard greens, cooked	1 cup	360 mg
sardines, canned	8 medium	350 mg
blackstrap molasses	2 tablespoons	280 mg
sesame seed meal (tahini)	¼ cup	270 mg
kale, cooked	1 cup	200 mg
salmon, canned with bones	3 ounces	170 mg
broccoli, cooked	1 stalk	160 mg
tofu (soybean curd)	4 ounces	150 mg
corn tortillas	2	120 mg
calcium-fortified orange juice	1 cup	320 mg

Also—when making soup stock from bones, add one or two tablespoons of vinegar during the boiling process. The acid in the vinegar will dissolve the calcium out of the bones, providing a soup stock unusually rich in calcium.

intake should have started many years earlier, to enable women to reach menopause with maximum bone strength. When estrogen levels drop off at menopause, bone loss is accelerated in most women. Calcium supplements started at this time have not been shown to protect the bones of the vertebral spine, but do have some protective effect on the long bones of the legs and arms. This protective effect is maximized if estrogen is also taken, as explained in Chapter 10.

Vitamin D must be present in the body to allow absorption of calcium from the intestine. This vitamin is formed on bare skin when we are outdoors in the sun. It is stored in the liver until needed. However, many people are cut off from the sun by clothing, remaining indoors, long dark winters, window glass, or smog. Others rightly fear that excess sun exposure may cause skin cancer or more rapid aging of skin. For these reasons Vitamin D has been added to many milk products; 8 ounces of fortified skim, low-fat, or whole milk provides 100 International Units (IU) of Vitamin D. Older women should get about 400 IU of Vitamin D daily to ensure optimum calcium absorption. This is most easily done by taking a daily multivitamin supplement containing Vitamin D. Excess Vitamin D (over 400 IU daily) is not advisable; this vitamin should be taken in "megadoses" only in a very few medical conditions.

A very high protein diet is one which contains twice the body's daily need for protein — ham and eggs for breakfast and meat, fish, poultry, or dairy products at other meals. Eating like this is common in Western countries; many people consider such food indispensable for health, and a symbol of good living. Dieters often subsist mainly on protein-rich foods. While small amounts of protein are essential, large amounts can cause problems. Animal foods are often high in fat and can lead to obesity and heart disease. In addition, they play a role in the osteoporosis story. The end products of digesting protein-rich foods are acids such as sulfuric acid, which the body excretes in the urine. In response, the kidneys excrete calcium to balance this acid. Even young people eating a very high protein diet lose significant amounts of calcium in their urine. The post-menopausal woman is most at risk from this dietary cause of calcium loss, because of her lack of estrogen with its protective effect on bones.

Bone studies on elderly women eating high-meat diets (the Eskimo), mixed diets (the average American), and vegetarian diets (Seventh-Day Adventists), show that high-meat eaters have the most osteoporosis, and vegetarians the least. Nutritional research indicates that the post-menopausal woman should not emphasize flesh foods, but concentrate on eating whole grains, beans, vegetables, fruits, and nonfat or low-fat milk products. In middle age and beyond, women and men will be healthier if they try new answers to the question, "What's for dinner?" Try some of these answers: baked potatoes and a big salad with bean sprouts and toasted sesame seeds, or split pea soup with whole wheat bread and cheese, or curried mixed vegetables with brown rice and yogurt. Sound good? Turn to Chapter 15 for further ideas.

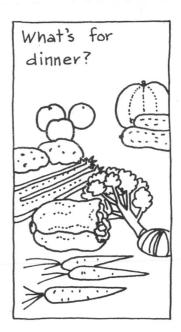

A diet high in salt (sodium chloride) is detrimental in several ways. It has long been known that too much salt can lead to high blood pressure in susceptible people. Recently it has also been found that salt has the effect of causing the kidneys to excrete more calcium in the urine. Over the long run such urinary loss of calcium can contribute to osteoporosis. Dramatic decreases in urinary calcium have been documented in patients with kidney stones when they reduce their salt intake.

Women who have never had children have more risk of osteoporosis, because the high hormone output in pregnancy contributes to bone strength. While this is true in western countries, where pregnancies are limited in number and dietary calcium is adequate, it is often not true in developing countries where numerous pregnancies and a poor diet can lead to bone weakness.

The relationship between heavy caffeine use and osteoporosis has only recently been studied. Caffeine is found in coffee, tea, colas and other soft drinks, and some medicines. In high doses caffeine can increase calcium loss from the body. This effect is small if a person drinks only one or two cups of coffee or tea daily, but can be significant if strong coffee or tea is consumed all day long. Since caffeine has other negative effects on health, contributing to chronic anxiety, disturbed sleep, and possibly to breast cysts, it is best to use it sparingly. Many heavy coffee drinkers are also smokers; these habits tend to be linked. Suggestions for quitting are discussed in Chapters 15 and 17.

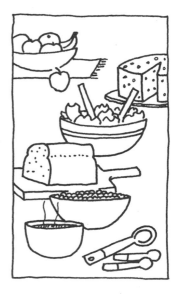

Estrogen and Osteoporosis

Osteoporosis can be prevented almost entirely by the use of estrogen tablets, beginning at the menopause and continuing for many years. Estrogen is very effective in halting the process of bone thinning and promoting bone strength. Numerous studies have shown a reduction in bone fractures among women taking estrogen tablets, and many doctors regard this medication as an important answer to the problem of bone loss with aging. Others, however, point out that every powerful medicine has some adverse side effects, and it is not safe or feasible to treat all women with hormones. Better ways are needed to identify those most at risk for fractures and, ideally, offer them a low dose of hormones combined with calcium and exercise.

Women who cannot take estrogen may use a progestin tablet regularly to help prevent osteoporosis. These compounds are not quite as effective as estrogen but do help to prevent bone loss and hot flashes. However, as explained in Chapter 10, their long-term side effects on the heart, blood vessels, and breasts need more study.

Some researchers suggest that women should take fluoride supplements to retard bone loss, along with varying amounts of calcium, vitamin D, and estrogen. Fluoride will help with the problem, but the suggested large doses have unacceptable toxicity and should not be used.

This has been a complex chapter because of the many factors that influence bone strength. In summary, some people are more at risk than others for fractures due to osteoporosis. As the table on page 56 shows, the woman most at risk is Asian or white, thin, with a family history of fractures with aging, and an early menopause. These genetic risks are greatly increased if she smokes, drinks heavily, does not exercise, and eats a high-protein, low-calcium diet. Conversely, women of any genetic background can greatly decrease their risk of fractures with aging by not smoking, exercising daily, eating high-calcium foods, taking calcium supplements with vitamin D, and minimizing meat, alcohol, salt, and caffeine in their diets. Finally, estrogen and progestin tablets can be taken after the menopause to prevent osteoporosis. The decision to take these hormones needs careful thought by a woman and her doctor because of their potential side effects, as discussed in Chapter 10. As soon as the pills are discontinued, the risk of bone loss returns. In any case, we never outgrow our need for healthy eating and body movement.

Janice, at 53, felt more secure after starting estrogen tablets to increase her bone strength. At 52 she had tripped on the street and fractured her ankle. The year before she broke her wrist when she fell on her stairs. Slim and small, Janice had followed a high-protein reducing diet for years. She had difficulty digesting milk products. She had a sedentary job in a bank and rarely exercised beyond doing housework. She was happy to take estrogen pills; they seemed the easiest solution and they also ended her hot flashes.

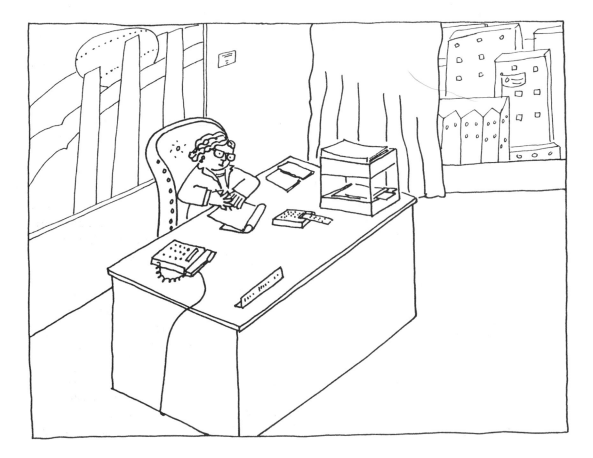

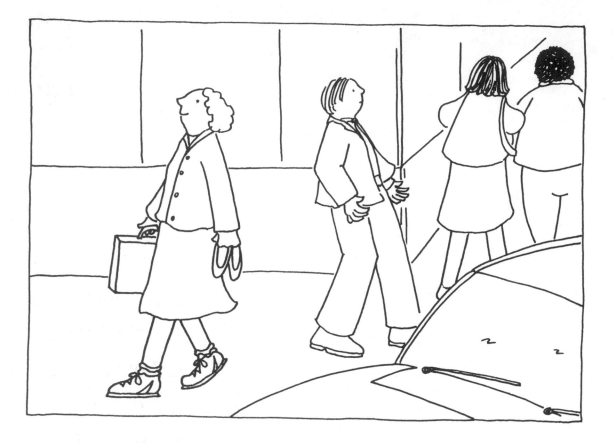

Ruth knew that she did not want to take hormones after the menopause. She always tried to find natural remedies for physical problems and was not a believer in pills. She was determined to see the menopause as a natural part of life, and not get upset by it. When her chiropractor told her she needed more exercise she began walking to and from work in tennis shoes. He also suggested that she chew mint-flavored calcium tablets after meals. She did some reading on the menopause and felt secure in her decision to let nature take its course.

Keep Your Bones Strong...How to Avoid Osteoporosis

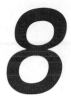

Popular mythology depicts the menopausal woman as going a little off her rocker. Are there special psychological risks for menopausal women? Are they more prone to depression, anxiety, irritability, and a general inability to cope?

If a woman in her late 40s gets angry or cries, her emotion is often blamed on "the change of life," just as in her 30s it was blamed on her periods or pregnancy. This kind of thinking can make women feel helpless, at the mercy of their hormones. It often prevents them from examining the factors in their relationships, families, or jobs that may well cause anger or depression.

Hormones and Psychology: Is Menopause a Time of Emotional Imbalance?

The group was talking about their emotional responses to the menopause. "The menopause has been really a hard time for me," said Sally. "I feel much more vulnerable and get depressed easily. I cry when my daughter leaves home or if my boss is unreasonable." "Listen, Sally," said Petra, "You're facing the classic mid-life crisis in my opinion. You'll be living alone when your daughter gets married and if your boss fires you you're sunk!" "It's too bad it all happens at once," answered Sally. "I have a hard time coping with hot flashes, my boss, and my daughter's leaving." "Something similar happened to me," said Alice. "Then I moved into a house with some friends and it got better. I wasn't lonely and my expenses went way down. Actually I feel happier than I have in years — and I'm going through the menopause too."

It is important to attempt to clarify the issues — do the end of ovulation and the drop in hormone levels at the menopause create a psychological imbalance in some women, triggering depression, anxiety, or delusional thinking? Or is the drop in hormone levels relatively neutral, psychologically speaking? Perhaps emotional upset during the menopause is caused by important coincidental changes in women's lives and the way middle age is viewed in our culture, rather than by hormonal changes.

These two views of the psychology of menopause have been debated for some time, and the issues are complex and interrelated. In this chapter we will look at both sides, and attempt to synthesize what is valuable in the two viewpoints.

It is important to say at the outset that no peak of emotional illness is found in the menopausal years. Surveys of women in their mid–40s to mid–50s show that hot flashes and night sweats are the only symptoms *directly* related to menopause. Other symptoms, such as depression, anxiety, headaches, or dizzy spells, occur in some women before, during, and after the menopause, without a peak at any specific age. Moreover, these symptoms tend to occur together; some women experience many such problems, while others have very few.

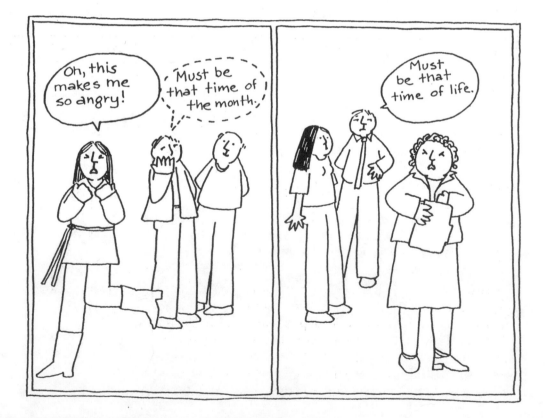

Hormones and Psychology: Is Menopause a Time of Emotional Imbalance?

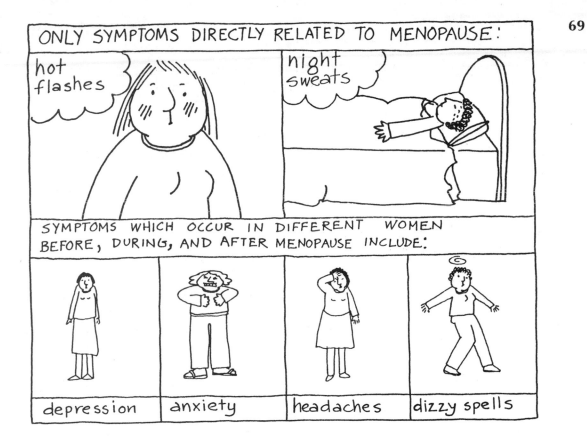

But what about women who *do* feel more anxious and depressed in their menopausal years? While they may be in the minority, how do we account for their problems, and what solutions are available? Can you predict whether you are more or less likely to experience this special kind of mid-life crisis?

Cultural Factors

Let's examine first the viewpoint of those who say it is *not* our hormones but our psychological reactions to aging and to outer circumstances that cause emotional problems in the menopause.

In our society women have been judged by their physical appearance more than anything else. The emphasis we place on beauty, fashion, figure, and youth makes it difficult for some women to value themselves as they become middle aged. This is especially true for those who used their glamour and sexiness to attract men and enhance their sense of self-esteem. It can be devastating for such a woman if her husband or lover leaves her for a younger mate, which sometimes happens in mid-life. Even without this problem she may become upset over vaginal dryness and pain with intercourse, feeling she is inadequate or invalidated as a sexual partner. She may feel that the end of her fertility means the end of her sexuality, and no longer view herself as a desirable person. She may consider hot flashes an embarrassing, visible sign of aging.

All these feelings can add up to anxiety and depression, which cause her to seek medical help. In most cases she will ask for or be given estrogen tablets, which are quite effective in relieving vaginal soreness with sex and reducing hot flashes. If this makes her feel better, we don't conclude that estrogen is an anti-depressant, but that the hormone relieved her physical symptoms, thereby providing her with a psychological lift.

Not all women react to aging with depression despite the cultural pressures that reward youthful female beauty and sexiness. Women who value themselves in their work, their avocations, or as friends or family members, have an easier time adjusting to the waning of youth. They may see the menopause as a welcome end to menstrual periods, and accept its bodily changes as normal. They go through the same hormonal process as the woman who becomes distraught, but they interpret it differently.

When children leave home for jobs, college, or marriage, some mothers have problems with this loss which they may blame on the menopause. Actually, this change can occur when a woman is in her 30s or her 60s, depending on when the youngest child leaves home. And despite all the mythology about the "empty nest," most parents feel quite positive about their children's maturity. Some women, however, do feel they have lost a major reason for existence — this is especially true of women who have focused their energies primarily on their children. Feelings of anxiety and depression about the loss of the mother role can be very painful. So can feelings of guilt about parenting, if children's lives are disturbed by illness, drugs, unwanted pregnancy, or failure in school or work.

If the woman's anxieties are blamed on the menopause, solutions are often sought in an estrogen pill or a tranquilizer and the real issue is left untouched. It is important for such women to reexamine what they want to do with their lives beyond mothering. They need to find new ways to express themselves which will raise their self-esteem. For this, a counselor or woman's group is more valuable than a pill.

Women who have interesting jobs, steady incomes, a sense of purpose, or things to do usually report fewer problems with the menopause. Conversely, women without as many options, in unskilled or poorly paid jobs, often view the menopause as more difficult. They may have less information about the physical symptoms of the menopause and react to them with more anxiety. Other unrelated illnesses may exist which compound the problem. The medical profession usually handles health problems with surgery, medicines, or tranquilizers, but frequently doesn't provide the kind of information and counseling that is needed to combat fears and years of negative stereotypes.

Cultural anthropologists who look at women's roles in various societies believe that the social context of our lives determines our reactions to aging. In our culture, the emphasis on youth and the nuclear family structure can make menopause a lonely time for women. In many other cultures, aging increases the status, power, and freedom that women experience; the menopausal years bring recognition and leadership roles in the extended family, ceremonies, and commerce. Freedom from sexual taboos allows women to travel more easily. Post-menopausal women are able to cultivate the more assertive side of their nature. Some of this can be seen in our own society if we look at older women who learn new skills, return to school, go into politics, or excel in their professions. What's expected of us often determines what we will be.

Hormonal Factors

Let's examine the opposite viewpoint, that many psychological problems in the menopause *are* directly related to decreasing estrogen levels. This is an unpopular stance with feminists, because it presents a picture of a woman as irrational and at the mercy of her hormones. It has also contributed to the widespread prescription of estrogen, tranquilizers, and antidepressant pills. Is there some validity to the viewpoint that emphasizes the chemistry of our inner environment over our reactions to the outside world?

Depression and anxiety, as well as positive mood states, are currently being studied from a biochemical perspective. The brain produces certain compounds that make us feel contented and euphoric, in response to exercise, food, love, meditation, and other stimuli. Other compounds in the brain can make us irritable and depressed. Some women experience marked mood shifts in relation to their hormonal changes, reporting tension before each menstrual period or depression after having a child. In fact, one in 500 women becomes so depressed or delusional after giving birth that she is said to have a postpartum psychosis.

During both menopause and giving birth there is a rapid drop in levels of estrogen and progesterone. It is possible that this shift may trigger depression in some susceptible people. Studies have been done to evaluate the role of estrogen replacement in the mental and emotional status of menopausal women. While the drug is not helpful with major depressions or psychoses, it has had beneficial effects on the moods of some women with more minor problems. Certain studies have shown that women with menopausal problems feel more cheerful, relaxed, and self-confident, and have improved memory and concentration after taking estrogen. Proponents of estrogen therapy feel that negative mental states may be directly caused by the menopause and alleviated by estrogen. Opponents think that any improvement seen with estrogen is due to the alleviation of hot flashes and night sweats, which secondarily improves mood by promoting sounder sleep and decreased anxiety about hot flashes.

It is difficult to resolve these questions with our present knowledge; there's probably truth in both positions. Our psychology — our moods, our outlook on life — is affected by the world around us *and* by our inner biology. The interactions among all these factors are so intimate that it is artificial to try to separate them. During the menopausal years the body goes through a major transition which is experienced differently by every woman, depending on her general health, her body awareness, and the rapidity of her hormone drop. Her psychological reaction to this transitional phase will be determined by both her biochemistry and her outer circumstances. Each affects the other — inner and outer worlds are inseparable, and in constant interaction.

Psychologists once proclaimed "biology is destiny" — meaning women were bound to go through certain predictable physical and emotional stages because of their reproductive systems. A more balanced viewpoint is that biology is only a part of destiny, along with the social environment in which we live.

Hormones and Psychology: Is Menopause a Time of Emotional Imbalance?

Moreover, as we understand this riddle we can direct at least some of our destiny by choosing to enhance our health and self-esteem.

Women reading this chapter may apply it individually according to their own experiences. Some will be pleased to discover that they need not become depressed or "go crazy" just because their periods stop. They need not experience the "raging imbalance of hormones" they have heard about. Other readers may feel that their emotional symptoms are intimately tied to their menopause, and will find relief in the knowledge that hormones can affect mood and emotions.

Menopausal women with physical or psychological problems are frequently given potent medications instead of the information and counseling they may need. Tranquilizers, sedatives, and antidepressants will only mask the issues, and should be avoided unless their use is really necessary for serious emotional problems. These drugs are often addicting and may have unpleasant side effects. Try counseling, exercise, relaxation techniques, and good nutrition first; the side effects of *these* measures make you feel

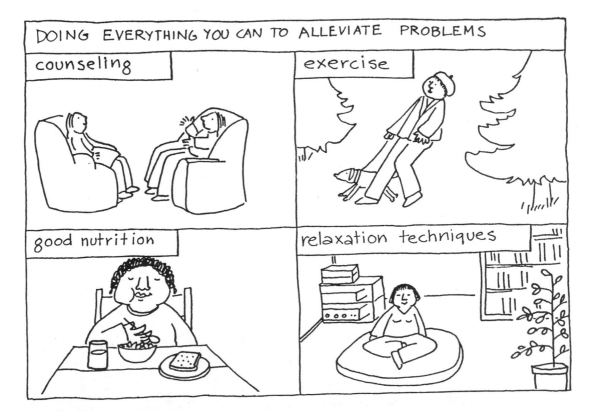

DOING EVERYTHING YOU CAN TO ALLEVIATE PROBLEMS

counseling

exercise

good nutrition

relaxation techniques

better, not worse. Sometimes what women need above all is to find — or establish — a self-help group of other mid-life women, to develop more positive images of the menopause and aging.

Some women may also want to try estrogen therapy for their physical and psychological symptoms. They should read Chapter 10 on the pros and cons of estrogen therapy, and evaluate their response to the medicine with understanding and caution.

Gail had a very hectic job and had gotten into the habit of taking tranquilizers to calm down. When she went through the menopause her gynecologist gave her estrogen and a progestin, and her internist gave her diuretics and tranquilizers. Her orthopedist gave her muscle relaxants. She drank a fair amount of coffee throughout the day and alcohol at night to calm down. One day as Gail stood in front of her medicine cabinet she knew something was wrong. She felt terrible inside, shaky and weak. She realized that she never allowed herself to feel the normal state of her body — she was always taking something to alter it. Her medicine cabinet became a blur of yellow, orange, green, and white pills. "I'm going to stop all these drugs," she heard herself say. Gail had a very uncomfortable time of it, and had to take a leave of absence from work, but she did manage to quit taking all pills. She found that acupuncture helped her withdrawal problems, as did a self-help group. Now she just has a hectic job, but no drug problem. "I like knowing what my body is going through," said Gail. "I'd rather have a hot flash or an anxious hour than be in a chemical fog."

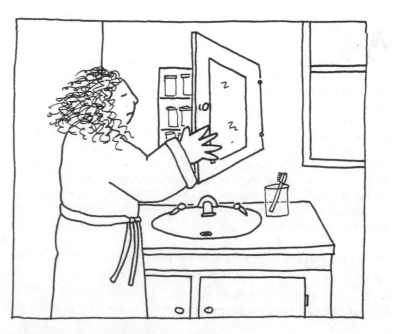

Hormones and Psychology: Is Menopause a Time of Emotional Imbalance?

9

*M*ary's periods became very light and far apart when she was 30. A few years later they disappeared entirely and she began having hot flashes. Mary lived in a rural mountainous part of the country and rarely went to the doctor. When she was hospitalized for a broken leg at 36 it was found that she had some osteoporosis, and blood tests revealed she was post-menopausal. Mary's doctor suggested that she take estrogens, a progestin at the end of each month, and daily calcium pills. She helped Mary understand the importance of taking these medicines and having yearly checkups. Mary was pleased that her hot flashes went away and she had no more pain with intercourse. She read a good book on the menopause and understood what had happened to her.

When Periods Stop Before 40

Menopause is considered early or premature if it occurs before the age of 40. The most common reason for early menopause is surgical removal of the uterus and ovaries, but occasionally a woman goes into natural menopause before 40. In this chapter we will look at both natural and surgical premature menopause, discuss the problems of this condition, and make recommendations for preserving health and sexuality despite the cessation of periods.

Conditions That Are Not Premature Menopause

When a woman in her 20s or 30s stops having menstrual periods there may be many reasons for it. Pregnancy, stress, or illness are common causes, and weight loss, prolonged strenuous exercise, or excessive weight gain can also play a role. Stopping the birth control pill may cause periods to cease for a year or more. Occasionally an excess of prolactin, the milk-promoting hormone of the pituitary, interrupts periods and causes milky fluid in the nipples. Thorazine[R]* and related drugs prescribed for severe emotional illness produce similar results.

Each of these conditions — none of which is premature menopause — needs to be considered when a woman's periods stop prematurely. Blood tests to diagnose premature menopause focus mainly on two hormones from the pituitary gland which stimulate the ovary to ovulate; they're called follicle-stimulating hormone (FSH) and luteinizing hormone (LH). When these hormones are low, the ovaries are temporarily at rest, but the woman is not menopausal. The pituitary gland and the ovaries will generally resume their activity when a woman's general health, emotional well-being, or hormone balance improves; the pituitary will put out more FSH and LH, the ovaries will be stimulated, and ovulation and menstruation will occur.

What Is Premature Menopause?

Sometimes the levels of FSH and LH are found to be very high. The ovaries are bombarded by stimuli but do not respond with ovulation, because the areas in the ovaries which produce egg

*Chlorpromazine is the generic name for Thorazine[R].

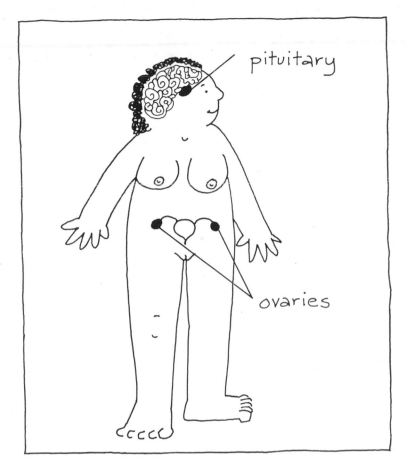

cells and estrogenic hormones are scarce and non-functional. This is premature menopause. Sometimes there is a genetic basis for this rare condition — the cells in the ovaries were programmed from birth to function for a shorter time because they were few in number or because of an abnormal gene. Another reason for premature menopause is that the woman develops antibodies to various glands in her body, such as her ovaries or her thyroid gland, thereby blocking glandular function. Women with premature menopause should have blood tests to check for such antibodies, for while there is no good treatment as yet for this problem, replacement hormones often make her feel more normal.

When premature menopause occurs in a woman's 30s, she usually gets hot flashes in the same way older women do. If it occurs even earlier, her symptoms may be less noticeable. Some young women have menstrual periods for only a few years — and they never experience hot flashes. The current explanation for this is that these women have never become accustomed to a high estrogen level, so they do not react to its withdrawal (see Chapter 4).

Pregnancy and Premature Menopause

Premature menopause can be extremely disappointing to the woman who wants to become pregnant. However, some women with a naturally occurring early menopause do conceive after hormone treatment. Those who desire pregnancy should consult a gynecologist who specializes in infertility problems. In some cases treatment with estrogen or other medicines will restore ovulation and fertility, at least for a time.

If pregnancy is not possible for the woman with premature menopause, she may want to consider adopting a baby. An excellent book on adoption is included in the book list on page 185.

Early Menopause from Surgery

Though naturally occurring premature menopause is rare, surgically induced early menopause is quite common in the United States today. About 25% of women who have hysterectomies under age 40 also have both ovaries removed. (If even one ovary is left in, the woman will continue to secrete estrogen and progesterone and will not experience menopausal symptoms until her late 40s or early 50s). Sometimes removing both ovaries is absolutely essential; overwhelming infection, tumors, cancer, severe endometriosis, or debilitating pelvic pain from scar tissue may leave no other course.

However, in some cases the ovaries are removed because the gynecologist has been taught they are not important once the uterus is removed. The argument against this view, and in favor of retaining the ovaries whenever possible, is discussed in Chapter 3. This crucial point requires open discussion with the doctor *before* pelvic surgery, so women can make informed choices.

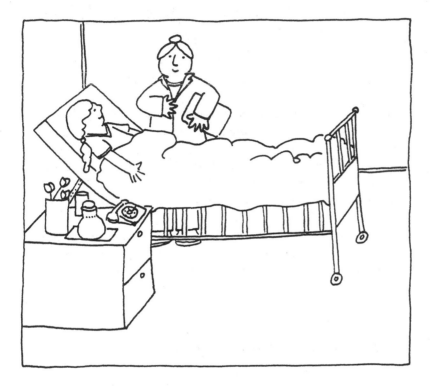

When Carolyn was 25 she developed a severe infection in her tubes and ovaries, possibly associated with an IUD she had been using. Despite hospitalization and antibiotics it was necessary to remove her uterus and both ovaries in order to control the infection. She was given estrogen pills to prevent the symptoms of premature menopause. Carolyn was very unhappy and resentful about what had happened to her. At one point a friend persuaded her to stop taking the estrogen and try megavitamins and herbal capsules, but she developed severe hot flashes and vaginal dryness whenever she did so. Ultimately she resolved to stay on estrogen until her mid-40s, and then taper the dose a bit. With time and counseling she regained a positive outlook, and pursued a career as a health professional. Later she married and adopted a baby.

If a young woman's ovaries are removed in surgery, she will undergo an abrupt premature menopause. She will not have the gradual decrease in estrogen experienced by women with natural menopause, so her symptoms may be more intense. Hot flashes can occur immediately after surgery unless estrogen replacement is started promptly. Most women with this condition decide to take estrogen tablets to prevent hot flashes and vaginal dryness. Others take estrogen for a time and then discontinue it because of side effects, fear of side effects, or the inconvenience of daily pill-taking.

What is the best advice for the woman with premature menopause? Should she take replacement hormones? What does she need to know in order to make a wise decision?

Replacement Hormones

Copying nature as closely as possible has many advantages in this situation. The ovaries normally secrete estrogen, progesterone, and androgens until age 50, and androgens thereafter into old age. Some of these androgens are converted to estrogen in body fat. The woman with premature menopause can duplicate this situation by taking a moderate dose of estrogen until her mid-40s, a lower dose until age 50, and a very small dose thereafter. If she has retained her uterus she should take a progestin along with the estrogen for the last part of each cycle, as explained in Chapter 10. These hormones will prevent hot flashes, vaginal dryness or soreness, and osteoporosis (see Chapter 7), which otherwise might begin earlier in life and cause fractures at a younger age.

Many women feel well on these replacement hormones and find that their sex drive is satisfactory. However, some women with premature menopause are quite distressed by a lowering of their sexual responsiveness at an age when other women are reaching their peak. If estrogen does not restore sexual interest, doctors can prescribe a low dose of testosterone by monthly injection (very rarely used in the United States) or in the form of 1% testosterone cream to be applied to the vaginal opening every other day in small amounts (see Chapter 3).

Women whose ovaries are removed by surgery before their normal menopause run a higher risk of having a heart attack later on. The reason for this is believed to be that the body's estrogen alters the levels and types of blood fats in a healthy way. When the ovaries are removed this protection is missing, but replacement estrogen in pill form can produce a similar effect, as discussed in Chapter 10.

In deciding to take estrogen, the woman with premature menopause is helping to prevent discomfort and long-term problems of heart and bone disease (osteoporosis); at the same time the medication may cause her some problems. No estrogen taken by mouth can exactly copy the complex ebb and flow of natural hormone secretions. The data on side effects from estrogen replacement are discussed in detail in the following chapter. Although most women with premature menopause do decide to take estrogens, some do not. For these women it is especially important to guard against osteoporosis and heart disease with exercise and good nutrition. They should exercise vigorously every day to keep their bones strong and promote cardiac fitness. They should not smoke or drink excess alcohol. They should eat a very low-fat, high-calcium diet without too much protein, to prevent osteoporosis. They would do well to consult a physician who is interested in preventive medicine, so they can monitor their levels of serum cholesterol and bone calcification.

These are the problems related to premature menopause, but there's an advantage on the other side of the equation: the risk of breast cancer is lessened! The earlier a woman experiences menopause, the less likely she is to develop breast cancer. Unfortunately, this reduced risk does not necessarily hold true for women on long-term estrogen replacement therapy (see Chapter 10).

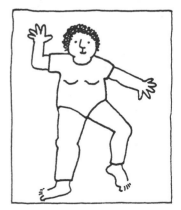

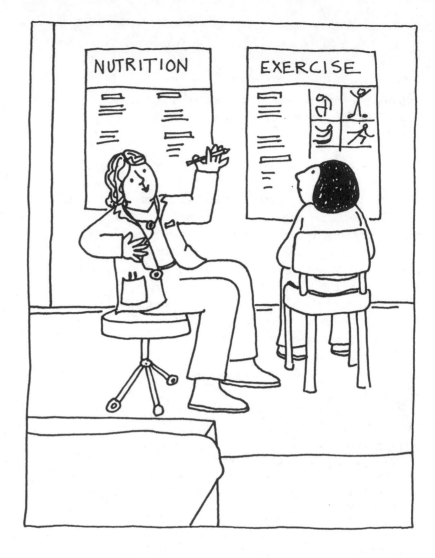

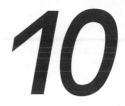

*No one ever told us we had to study our lives, make of our lives a
study, as if learning natural history.*

— Adrienne Rich

*T*he women in the group were discussing estrogen. *"After I talked
to my doctor I felt like I'd shrivel up totally if I didn't take it," said
Wendy. "Then I read 'Women and the Crisis in Sex Hormones' and
decided to take Vitamin E and ginseng." "I don't feel I need anything
as powerful as estrogen," said Roberta. "I've been thinking about how
to stay healthy and it doesn't make sense to keep putting an artificial
hormone into my body. Besides, my daughter's always reminding me
about all the side effects they've discovered about the pill." Finally
Carol spoke up: "It's been really important for me to take estrogen. It's
made me feel much better mentally and physically. And I'm so glad to
be rid of hot flashes and be able to sleep through the night." "I wish
there was a lot more research on this question," said Clara. "I'm going
to wait until I see better evidence in support of estrogen, and by then
I'll probably be too old to care one way or the other." "Billions for outer
space, pennies for inner," sighed Wendy.*

Estrogen Replacement Therapy: The Pros, Cons, and Unknowns

Amazing advances in chemistry and pharmacology in our
time have created many new choices for doctors and patients.
Common discomforts and aging itself are no longer accepted as

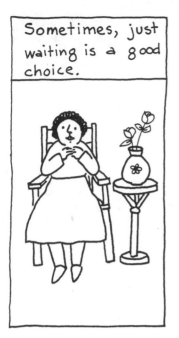

Sometimes, just waiting is a good choice.

inevitable. Instead they are combatted with medicines and procedures, some very helpful — and others potentially dangerous. We must all tackle the difficult chore of choosing reasonably among the possible therapies for our problems. Sometimes just waiting is a good choice, and sometimes treatment is necessary. The menopausal woman's choice about using estrogen or not is especially problematic, because the therapy is relatively new, controversial, and non-essential, yet quite helpful to some. The benefits and risks of taking estrogen — and not taking it — vary from person to person. In this chapter we will look at the pros, cons, and unknowns of estrogen therapy in some detail. The following chapter summarizes the information more briefly, and provides a self-rating scale to help you make a careful decision, together with your doctor.

A Little History

Since the beginnings of human evolution, women have gone through the menopause without taking hormones. It's true that surviving at all to middle age was once pretty rare, but for cen-

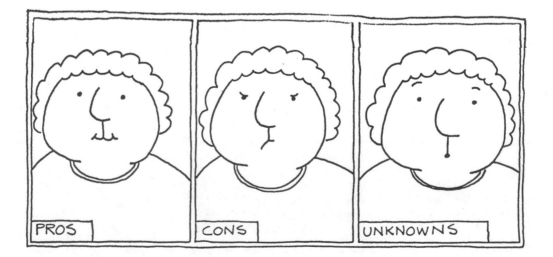

PROS | CONS | UNKNOWNS

turies many people have lived to old age, women often outliving men. In places where many women and men live today to be 100 — remote mountainous areas in Ecuador, Pakistan, or southern Russia — the use of estrogen therapy is certainly very low! Extreme longevity seems to depend not on any drug therapy, but on a favorable family history and a lifestyle characterized by exercise, moderate eating and drinking, and an optimistic attitude.

When estrogen was first isolated in the 1920s, it was used for women who had lost their ovaries through surgery, as well as for women with severe problems after natural menopause. However, its use was not widespread until the 1960s, when a book entitled *Feminine Forever,* by Robert Wilson, popularized estrogen use for all women who wanted to retard aging and retain their feminine allure. The use of "estrogen replacement therapy," or ERT, spread widely among middle- and upper-class women treated by private physicians. Women wanted ERT because they were told they would age more slowly, look more attractive, and avoid the discomforts of menopause. Many doctors promoted ERT because it was a powerful and effective new treatment that provided an apparently quick answer to problems that were hard to deal with, like hot flashes, insomnia, vaginal soreness, mid-life crises, and depression. While the drug does deal with the first three problems, it does not necessarily solve the social and psychological difficulties of the middle years. Helping a patient clarify such problems through counseling takes more time than the average doctor can spare, so prescriptions are often written as an alternative.

Another interested party in this use of estrogens has been the drug companies which manufacture the multitude of pills, injections, and creams designed for menopausal women. Thirty to forty million women in the United States today are post-menopausal. In some middle-class areas, more than half the post-menopausal women used ERT in 1975.

In the mid-1970s reports began to appear linking estrogen use in post-menopausal women to cancer of the uterus. Women were found to be about five times more likely to develop this cancer if they used estrogen replacement therapy. There was a rapid decline in the prescription of ERT after these reports, and this decline lasted several years. Recently, however, new studies show that the addition of a progestin for 10 to 14 days at the end of each 25-day course of estrogen protects women quite effectively against uterine cancer. As this reassuring news became known, doctors began to prescribe post-menopausal hormones again quite liberally.

It has been said that widespread use of the birth control pill by young women represents an unprecedented sociomedical experiment. Never before in human history has a powerful medicine been taken so widely by healthy persons to achieve a goal — contraception — that could be met in other ways. The widespread use of ERT represents a similar sociomedical experiment. Never before in human history has a large proportion of aging women taken medicines to prolong the youthful hormonal state of the reproductive years into the 50s and 60s and beyond. This alteration of the natural plan for the human body may have both benefits and risks, which need to be uncovered by painstaking study. Some questions about the effects of ERT are being answered, some are still being debated. What are the types of hormones currently available and their advantages and disadvantages?

Estrogen:
Types and Methods of Use

Estrogens that occur naturally in people are of three types: estrone, estradiol, and estriol. Chemical variations of these three forms are used as medicines, and their differing actions and potencies are debated among pharmacologists. Dosage and the method of administration also affect women's responses to particular estrogens.

Most estrogen tablets currently on the market in the U.S. are composed of various forms of estrone or estradiol. Estradiol is the principal estrogen naturally present in women before the menopause; estrone is the main estrogen present after menopause. Estrone and estradiol are very similar and each can be converted into the other within the body. Estriol is a weak estrogen created by the placenta and the breakdown of other estrogens in the body. It is not currently available in the U.S. in pill form, but it is used in some other countries.

The most commonly prescribed estrogen in the U.S. today is conjugated equine estrogen, available generically* and under the brand name Premarin (Ayerst Laboratories). It is a mixture of estrone and other forms of estrogen. It's popular because it is "natural," derived from pregnant mares' urine, rather than synthesized in the laboratory. However, there is no real evidence for or against the use of conjugated equine estrogens as opposed to other estrogen products currently on the market, such as Ogen (Abbott), Estrace (Mead Johnson Pharmaceutical), or their generic equivalents, when available. See the table on page 88.

In my opinion, women should not take any estrogen which is combined with a tranquilizer, such as Menrium (Roche), which contains Librium, or PMB (Ayerst Laboratories), which contains meprobamate. Librium and meprobamate cause sedation and can be habit forming. Experts believe that tranquilizers should be used only when absolutely necessary for anxiety, and never given with a drug designed for daily administration. Menopausal women should probably avoid taking the so-called non-steroidal estrogens, such as DES (diethylstilbestrol — Lilly) or TACE (Merrell Dow), because of the association of these drugs with vaginal cancer in the female children of women who took the medicines in pregnancy. The non-steroidal estrogens are chemically less similar to natural estrogens, and need further safety evaluation.

Estrogen is also available in adhesive patches which are applied to the skin of the abdomen or thigh (Estraderm — Ciba-Geigy). The hormone is gradually and evenly absorbed through the skin over a 3½ day period. The patches are changed twice a week, but the woman is free to bathe or swim at any time. There

---

* Most drugs have an official or generic name, and also one or more trade names given by different manufacturing companies. You will pay less for a prescription written with the generic name than for one with a well known trade name. However, you may get a medicine of lower quality, depending on the standards of the manufacturer. Confer with your doctor and pharmacist about this.

Table of Commonly Prescribed Estrogens (generic equivalents are often available)

Brand Name	Generic Name	Tablet Strength	Comments
Estrace	estradiol	1 mg,* 2 mg*	
Estraderm	estradiol	.05 mg, .1 mg	Estraderm, a skin patch, releases estrogen into the blood stream.
Ogen	estropipate (estrone)	.625 mg,* 1.25 mg,* 2.5 mg,* 5 mg*	
Premarin	conjugated estrogens	.3 mg, .625 mg, .9 mg, 1.25 mg, 2.5 mg	Premarin and its generic equivalents are the most commonly prescribed estrogens in current use.
Premarin with methyl-testosterone	conjugated estrogens (E) + methyltestosterone (T)	.625 mg E + 5 mg T 1.25 mg E + 10 mg T	Regular use of oral testosterone may cause masculinization and and health problems. Not recommended.
Menrium	esterified estrogens (E) + chlordiazepoxide (Librium)	.2 mg E + 5 mg Librium .4 mg E + 5 mg Librium .4 mg E + 10 mg Librium	Librium, a tranquilizer, may be habit forming. Avoid any fixed combination of tranquilizers with estrogen.
PMB	conjugated estrogens (E) + meprobamate (M)	.45 mg E + 200 mg M .45 mg E + 400 mg M	Meprobamate, a tranquilizer, can be habit forming. Avoid any fixed combination of tranquilizers with estrogen.
DES	diethylstilbestrol	.1 mg, 1 mg, 5 mg	Not enough is known about the effects and doses of these synthetic estrogens to recommend their use. See text.
TACE	chlorotrianisene	12 mg, 25 mg, 72 mg	

* When this mark (*) follows a dose it means the tablet is scored and can easily be divided in half.

may be significant advantages and disadvantages to using estrogen by skin patch compared to the usual tablet form. When estrogen is taken by tablet it is absorbed through the intestinal tract and travels immediately to the liver, where it stimulates the production of a substance which causes high blood pressure in some individuals. Since estrogen by skin patch avoids this step it seems to be preferable for women prone to blood pressure problems. On the other hand, there is concern that estrogen absorbed through the skin may not have the same favorable effect on blood cholesterol that is found with oral tablets. More study is needed on these questions.

Estraderm patches come in two strengths, .05 mg and .1 mg. In most cases the lower strength, .05 mg, is sufficient.

Use of a Progestin with Estrogen

Estrogen used alone after the menopause has been associated with an increased risk of uterine cancer. This risk can be greatly reduced or eliminated by adding a progestin tablet daily to the last 10 to 14 days of the cycle. Progestins are compounds similar to progesterone, normally secreted by the ovaries after ovulation and in pregnancy. Natural progesterone is less effective when taken orally, but progestins can be taken in tablet form. It is extremely important that any woman who still has her uterus use the following kind of schedule if she wishes to take ERT. She should take an estrogen pill from the first to the 25th day of the month. She should also take a progestin from the 14th to the 25th day. Then she should stop taking both tablets for 5 or 6 days, and at this point she will usually have some bleeding. The progestin tablet has the effect of allowing the uterine lining to be evenly shed when all hormones are stopped. If the lining is sloughed off this way every month, it is much less likely that it will become cancerous.

If the woman's uterus has been removed by surgery, she should take a few days off estrogen each month, but she need not take a progestin. Any woman who has a uterus, however, should take a progestin whenever she takes daily estrogen. The addition

Table of Commonly Prescribed Progestin Tablets
(generic equivalents are often available)

Brand Name	Generic Name	Tablet Strength	Comments
Amen	medroxyprogesterone acetate	10 mg	The lowest dose that protects against uterine cancer is not known as yet.
Provera	medroxyprogesterone acetate	2.5 mg, 5 mg, 10 mg	
Norlutin	norethindrone	5 mg	
Norlutate	norethindrone acetate	5 mg	½ tablet is probably a sufficient dose to protect against uterine cancer.
Aygestin	norethindrone acetate	5 mg	

All tablets in this table are scored and can easily be divided in half.

of a progestin is also a good idea for a woman who has taken estrogen alone in the past and is no longer taking it. A 10-day course of a progestin will help her get rid of any excess uterine lining that might have built up. Some doctors prescribe a progestin even if estrogen has never been taken, especially in women who seem to produce abundant natural estrogen after the menopause. This occurs more often in women who have considerable body fat.

Adding a progestin to the estrogen cycle greatly reduces the risk of uterine cancer, but it also has disadvantages. Progestin compounds in the birth control pill were found to cause changes in the body's use of starches and sugars similar to the changes of diabetes, and to alter blood fats in an unfavorable way. They were implicated, along with estrogen, in high blood pressure, heart disease, and stroke. These risks must be balanced against the danger of uterine cancer. This kind of comparison needs to be made and individualized for each woman, based on her personal and family medical history.

Progestins currently on the market include Amen (Carnick), Provera (Upjohn), Norlutin, Norlutate (Parke-Davis), and

Aygestin (Ayerst). See the table on opposite page. Other progestins are available in birth control pills, but not for the postmenopausal woman. Research is needed to clarify the differences among these compounds in terms of side effects and to determine the lowest effective dose.

Labeling and Packaging of ERT Medicines

Women who take estrogens will note that an educational leaflet comes with each prescription informing patients about the risks and benefits of ERT. In this pamphlet they are told that estrogen is generally prescribed cyclically — three weeks on, one week off each month — to avoid overstimulation of the uterus. They are also told of the increased risk of cancer of the uterus with estrogen use, as well as other side effects. However, they are not told that most doctors are now prescribing a progestin during the last 10 to 14 days of estrogen therapy each month to decrease this cancer risk.

When women fill a prescription for a progestin they also are given an educational leaflet by the pharmacist, but this one only informs them of the dangers of taking progestins during pregnancy. No information on the use of this medicine after the menopause is included.

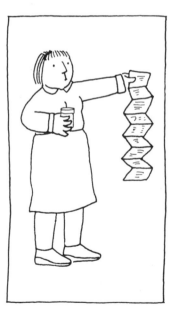

The U.S Food and Drug Administration (FDA) recommended in 1986 that estrogen manufacturers inform doctors that the use of a progestin at the end of an estrogen cycle is useful to prevent uterine hyperplasia — a precursor of uterine cancer. However, the FDA was not ready to endorse progestin use as a proven preventative of uterine cancer, and also noted that progestins have possible additional risks relating to levels of fats and sugars in the body. Because more research information is needed on these questions, there is no clear consensus from the FDA and drug companies as to what to say to the consumer. In the meantime, physicians and their patients are left with a confusing situation. Despite this hesitancy by the FDA, most doctors go ahead and prescribe a progestin along with estrogen whenever the woman has her uterus, to help prevent uterine cancer.

Reasons for Taking
Post-Menopausal Estrogens

Let's review the reasons women and their doctors favor using estrogens, and the dosages appropriate in each situation. Women under the age of 45 who have had a surgical menopause should review Chapter 9 before reading this section.

Hot flashes

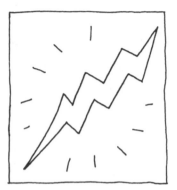

Estrogen will act rapidly to reduce this problem. The lowest dose that will prevent discomfort is the goal, and therefore women should keep a record of their hot flashes and start with the lowest dose of estrogen available. For some currently marketed products these doses are: Premarin (Ayerst) .3 mg, Ogen (Abbott) .3 mg (obtained by dividing the .625 mg tablet), and Estrace (Mead Johnson) .5 mg (obtained by dividing the 1 mg tablet).

These estrogen tablets are usually quickly effective in reducing distress from hot flashes. However, the symptom generally returns when estrogen is stopped. Taking estrogen, therefore, does not cure hot flashes but it does postpone them until the time that ERT is stopped. Some women elect to take ERT indefinitely and thus may never have hot flashes. Other women take estrogen for temporary relief of hot flashes and then decide to stop it after a few months or a few years. Since the mechanisms involved in hot flashes are related to rapid decrease in estrogen levels (see Chapter 4), the best way to cease estrogen therapy is to taper off very slowly. The woman taking .625 mg of conjugated estrogens can switch to .3 mg daily for a month or two, then take this dose every other day, and finally stop it entirely. She should continue with a progestin in the second half of each cycle unless her uterus has been removed. Sometimes after a three-to-six-month trial of this regimen, hot flashes will be lessened. If not, the woman can resume estrogen and repeat the tapering-off process when she is ready. Many women find they can cope with the problem of hot flashes when they gradually and slowly reduce the estrogen dose this way.

If estrogens cannot be used, some doctors use injectable or oral progestins alone to relieve hot flashes. These medications are not as effective as estrogens, but do help in many cases. However, they can cause irregular vaginal bleeding, depression, weight gain, and possible long-term side effects on the heart and blood vessels. Their use should be limited, therefore, to special patients who do not respond to other measures.

Vaginal soreness

Insertion of a penis, fingers, or a vaginal speculum can be uncomfortable or painful in post-menopausal women, because estrogen and androgen secretion from the ovaries has decreased. One action of these hormones is to keep the vaginal lining cells thickened and resistant to friction. When hormone levels drop, this cellular layer becomes thinner, drier, and less elastic. The vagina is then more likely to be sore or irritated by penetration. This situation can be alleviated by oral estrogen tablets, but also by the use of a low-dose estrogen cream. Some women who do not want to take estrogen orally use a hormonal cream very successfully.

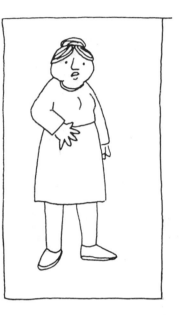

If a woman is taking oral estrogen, even in the smallest doses, she will generally not need to use vaginal estrogen creams. The low-dose cream treatment advocated in this section is designed for women who want to alleviate vaginal soreness without taking other forms of ERT.

One of the commonly used estrogen creams is Premarin cream. This comes with an applicator calibrated for 1 to 4 grams of cream; the dose frequently suggested is 2 to 4 grams daily or one-half to one applicator applied vaginally. As there is .625 mg of Premarin per gram of the cream, this dose would give a woman 1.25 to 2.5 mg of estrogen daily. The estrogen is rapidly absorbed from the vagina. In fact, estrogen cream in high doses can be stronger than pills, as hormones from the cream enter the blood stream directly and are not subject to the digestive process.

However, lower doses of estrogen cream than currently suggested by most doctors and drug companies are effective. A recent British study showed that vaginal soreness responds to as little as .1 mg of estrogen daily in cream, an amount taking up slightly less than one-eighth inch in the applicator. Clearly the applicator needs to be redesigned or the cream reformulated to a lower concentration. In the meantime, women should look at a Premarin applicator very carefully and notice there are five small rings in the plastic between the 1-gram mark and the top of the

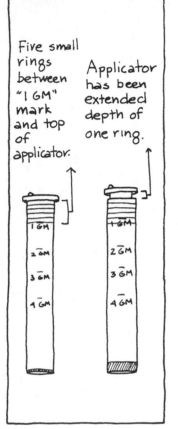

Five small rings between "1 GM" mark and top of applicator.

Applicator has been extended depth of one ring.

applicator (see illustration). The distance between two of those rings will deliver about one-eighth inch of the cream. Some women need twice this amount (two to three rings or about one-fourth inch of cream) for the first 7 days of use in order to reach an acceptable level of comfort.

The cream should be directed towards the sore area which is usually inside the inner vaginal lips right at the entrance to the vagina. Apply the cream to that area with the applicator or with a finger, being sure to get to the sorest point. After 5 to 10 days of such treatment, the problem of pain with penetration is usually resolved. Thereafter, most women then use the cream every 2 or 3 days. Do not use the cream right before intercourse; it is designed for vaginal treatment, and not as a lubricant.

One study suggested that after about a week of estrogen cream use with these very low doses, the vaginal cells seem to erect a partial barrier to the systemic absorption of estrogens, so that no increased blood levels of estrogen were found. More research is needed to clarify the systemic effects of the very low doses of cream required to relieve vaginal discomfort.

Other estrogen creams besides Premarin may be used, following the same suggestions for lower dosage. Most are effective after a week of daily use of only a very small amount of cream (one-eighth to one-fourth inch). See the table on page 98.

When such small doses are used, is there a risk of uterine cancer? Probably not; but to be safe, some doctors recommend the use of a progestin for 10 days after a few months of cream use, and every 6 months thereafter.

The use of these minimal doses of estrogen cream eliminates most of the pain of vaginal penetration. However, it does not restore as much vaginal lubrication as was present before the menopause, so it's wise to use an oil or cream for lubrication during intercourse.

Androgen cream, which a pharmacist can make up as 1% or 2% testosterone in a water-soluble base, is also effective in preventing vaginal soreness after the menopause. It is used in the same way as estrogen cream; after a week or so of daily application, minimal amounts are effective twice weekly. No studies have been published that compare the use of estrogen and androgen creams; more research is needed in this area.

As Chapter 7 spells out, estrogen therapy retards the loss of calcium from bones after the menopause. Since ERT results in a lower rate of hip and forearm fractures and height loss, doctors often suggest women most at risk of osteoporosis begin ERT after the menopause and continue it for the rest of their lives. If ERT is stopped at any point, the bones begin to lose its beneficial effects.

We don't know the exact dose of ERT needed to prevent bone fractures. Probably protection increases with increasing dosages, but some benefit is derived even from small amounts. Most doctors are prescribing .625 mg of Premarin (Ayerst) and Ogen (Abbott), or 1 mg of Estrace (Mead Johnson), with a progestin at the end of each cycle (if the uterus is present). Recent research shows that half the usual dose of Premarin, or .3 mg, combined with a calcium intake of 1,500 mg daily through the diet or supplements, is also protective against bone loss. More work is needed to clarify this question of the lowest effective doses of estrogen in the long term prevention of brittle bones. In the meantime, remember that all mid-life women, including those on estrogen, need to get daily exercise and an increased calcium intake to keep their bones strong.

What ERT Won't Do

Though ERT has been shown to be helpful with hot flashes, vaginal soreness, and osteoporosis, it has *not* been proven to be helpful in preventing wrinkles or other signs of aging, or treating psychological problems. The effects of ERT on the heart and circulation are variable and complex; some studies show a protective effect, and others show increased risk. These data are summarized later in this chapter.

ERT is not designed to correct hormonal imbalances in menstruating women. It should generally not be taken until periods have stopped completely, because while they continue, the ovaries are producing natural estrogen. Before the menopause a progestin sometimes helps regulate bleeding problems.

Reasons for Not Taking
Post-Menopausal Estrogens

Cancer of the uterus

The main reason many women stopped ERT after 1975 was the finding that the medication increased the risk of developing uterine cancer. Fortunately, the cancers occurring in 95% of these women responded well to hysterectomy and other treatments. Subsequently it has been found that the use of a progestin in the second half of each estrogen cycle allows for complete shedding of the uterine lining and very substantially reduces the risk of uterine cancer. Some studies suggest that the risk of uterine cancer is even *lower* among estrogen and progestin users than among women who take no ERT at all.

The cancer risk remains, however, because some doctors do not prescribe a progestin for an adequate time each month (10 to 14 days) and some women neglect to take it. Since the FDA has not fully endorsed this use of progestins, as explained on page 91, patients are not yet regularly informed about it in the package inserts produced by drug companies.

Obesity also increases the risk of uterine cancer because of the increased amount of natural estrogen formed in the body's fat cells. Menopausal women who are more than 25 or 30 pounds overweight are not advised to take estrogen in most cases. They *should* take a 10-day course of a progestin to promote a shedding of the uterine lining which protects against this type of cancer. If bleeding occurs, some doctors suggest that they repeat the progestin every few months until there is no further bleeding.

Liver and gallbladder disease

As a rare complication, the birth control pill induces liver tumors. It is therefore wise for doctors to check for liver enlargement in women using ERT.

Women with liver disease due to alcohol or other causes should take no unnecessary medications, including ERT. Women taking estrogens have been found in several studies to have an increased risk of gallbladder disease. They require surgical removal of the gallbladder more than twice as often as other women. Gallbladder surgery is a major operation that can present significant risks to older women; a recent study shows the risk of dying after gallbladder surgery late in life is greater than the risk of dying after a hip fracture. Women most at risk for gallstones are those who are obese, have a high cholesterol dietary intake or blood level, or have diabetes, Crohn's disease, or some other rare illnesses. Native American women from the Southwest frequently develop gallstones. Any woman who has these risks or knows she has gallstones should avoid ERT, and should consume foods high in fiber (whole grains, beans, and vegetables) and very low in fat.

Depression

While some post-menopausal women have found that estrogen improves their mood, others find they are depressed by it, or by the added progestin. Such depression is sometimes related to an increased need for B vitamins, and is improved by the daily use of a B-complex pill containing 25 mg of vitamin B_6. If depression persists unrelated to any obvious factors in daily life, women can try stopping ERT to assess differences in their moods.

Uterine fibroids

Uterine fibroids are benign overgrowths of muscular tissue which enlarge the uterus. They are stimulated by estrogen, which explains why fibroids sometimes grow with the birth control pill or in pregnancy. Ordinarily fibroid tumors shrink after the menopause because of decreased estrogen levels and are rarely any further problem. However, ERT may cause continued growth of these tumors. Sometimes fibroids grow to a size that is uncomfortable and hysterectomy is suggested; it is safer and easier to avoid ERT if fibroids are growing.

Increased visits to physicians

Women who take ERT generally visit their physicians more frequently for routine checkups. It is a good idea for them to have a blood pressure and breast examination twice a year and an overall physical exam with blood chemistry determination

Table of Estrogen and Testosterone Vaginal Creams
(generic equivalents are often available)

Brand Name	Generic Name	Strength	Comments
Ogen cream	estropipate (estrone)	1.5 mg per gram of cream	
Premarin cream	conjugated estrogens	.625 mg per gram of cream	Use very small amount as explained in text, page 93.
Estrace cream	estradiol	.1 mg per gram of cream	
DES suppositories	diethylstilbestrol	.1 mg, .5 mg	
DV cream	dienestrol	.5 mg per applicator	DES and dienestrol are synthetic estrogens. Not enough is known about their effects and dosages, not recommended.
DV suppositories		.7 mg per suppository	
Testosterone cream	testosterone proprionate	1% or 2% in vanishing cream base	Must be made by pharmacist; generic only.

yearly. If they experience any vaginal bleeding at times other than the five days they are off the pills, they should have a biopsy or D&C to test the uterine lining.

These are recommendations for more medical care than the usual pattern for post-menopausal women. Ideally, older women should visit a doctor or nurse practitioner yearly for exams and screening tests, but many fail to do so after their reproductive years and seek care only for illness. On the one hand, more frequent visits may result in earlier recognition of abnormalities. On the other hand, they are costly, time-consuming, and result in more medical tests, surgeries, and drugs, some of which may be harmful.

Daily pill-taking and monthly periods

Many people dislike taking pills regularly. Women using ERT to prevent osteoporosis are counseled to continue it for the rest of their lives, but they may become bored or forgetful with this regimen. Others dislike it because they continue to have monthly

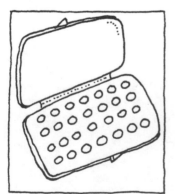

periods at an age when they had expected freedom from this function. The expense of daily pill use may be a financial burden to some women.

Controversies in ERT

The two areas where ERT is most controversial today are cardiovascular disease and breast cancer. Some research claims that ERT causes or worsens these conditions, while other studies show no effects or even benefits. When controversy prevails, it usually means the answers are complex and the right questions may not yet have been asked. Here's the currently available evidence.

Heart attacks, strokes, and high blood pressure

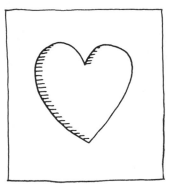

Since heart disease is the leading cause of death in older women, it is important to know the effects of ERT on the heart and blood vessels. However, at present the evidence is contradictory, with most studies showing a reduction in risk for high blood pressure and heart attack when women use ERT, and others showing the opposite.

Some of the claims made for the beneficial effects of estrogen on circulatory diseases such as heart attack and stroke come from studies with an obvious statistical flaw. Users of estrogen are compared to non-users in terms of death from circulatory disease, and estrogen users seem to do better. However, the studies ignore the fact that doctors tend to suggest estrogen to their healthier patients, and to discourage the use of hormones in women who already have risk factors such as obesity, high blood pressure, chest pains, diabetes, or heavy use of tobacco or alcohol. The population of women taking estrogen is therefore not comparable to the population not taking it; estrogen users are more health conscious from the beginning. When such women are followed for 5 or 10 years, it appears that they have lower risks of death from circulatory disease. This may be due to their good health habits, their estrogen use, or both. We do not know what weight to give to these various factors.

Part of the confusion about hormones and heart disease may stem from the fact that most studies have involved women on different types and dosages of estrogen, to which a week or two of progestin may or may not have been added. Experts in this field are currently saying that estrogen alone, in low doses, provides some protection against heart disease. Estrogen use results in lower levels of total serum cholesterol, and somewhat higher amounts of a fraction of cholesterol called HDL cholesterol that protects against blood vessel damage. However, the progestin added to estrogen at the end of each month is believed to act in the other direction, increasing the risk of blood vessel damage, stroke, and heart attack, by altering the type of fats in the blood stream in an unfavorable way.

It is ironic that progestins, so effective in preventing uterine cancer, may have a negative effect on the circulatory system. Women who have had a hysterectomy and therefore do not need added progestin may derive some protection from heart disease by using ERT. But women who have their uterus face a situation in which the benefits of estrogen on the heart and blood vessels are at least partially cancelled out by the progestin.

The effects of ERT on high blood pressure and stroke are also not conclusive. While the birth control pill in younger women has been shown to cause high blood pressure in some, this has not been a notable effect of ERT in post-menopausal women. But be cautious. Women taking ERT should have blood pressure checks every six months and stop hormones if the pressure rises significantly. If severe headaches develop while taking ERT, or if a woman notices any unusual symptoms, such as blurred vision, weakness, or numbness of any body part, or unusual pain in the chest or other area, she should stop her pills and seek medical attention. Women who are susceptible to blood pressure problems should consider the estrogen skin patch if they wish to take ERT (see p. 87–89).

All women using ERT, with or without progestin, should have periodic checks of their blood glucose and cholesterol. Everyone over 50 can diminish the risk of heart disease by following a lifestyle with lots of exercise and a low-fat, low-salt diet, as discussed in Chapters 14 and 15.

Studies aimed at determining whether ERT changes the risk of breast cancer show mixed results. Some are reassuring, but others show increased risk after long term use. While some researchers feel there is little association between the use of ERT and the subsequent development of breast cancer, others think estrogen may be a promoting factor for this disease. The risk appears to rise with the dose of hormones used, and the length of time they are taken. Other risk factors for breast cancer include the finding of "atypical proliferative" cells in a breast biopsy (just having lumpy breasts without these abnormal cells is not a risk factor), a family history of breast cancer, not having borne children or having your first child late in life (the earlier you bear a child, the more protection you have), and obesity. Women who were given DES (diethylstilbestrol) during pregnancy to prevent miscarriage show a small increased risk of breast cancer beginning 20 years later. In addition, several dietary factors have been implicated in breast cancer, such as a high content of fat, protein, or overall calories in the diet, and the use of alcohol. Recent studies have shown a possible connection between even moderate alcohol use (three drinks a week) and breast cancer, with increased risks for heavier drinkers. See Chapter 15 for more details.

At present our knowledge in this area is incomplete, which leaves women and their doctors in a dilemma. It is prudent advice for most women to use ERT in the lowest possible dose if they do decide to take it. Women should do breast self-exams monthly, be checked by a clinician every 6 months, and stop ERT if breast lumps develop, even if they are benign. Mammography (x-rays of breast tissue) should be performed every year in women over 50, and every other year between 40 and 50. Having mammograms regularly is important whether or not you take ERT, since they can detect very small abnormalities that cannot be felt on breast exam alone. Safe new techniques of visualizing body tissue, such as nuclear magnetic resonance (NMR), may also prove helpful in the detection of breast cancer.

Breast cancer is justifiably a major worry among mid-life women. It is important for all women to examine their breasts regularly and to seek medical care promptly if a breast lump is discovered. It is helpful to do breast exams lying down — in bed at night or in the bathtub. Remember that most lumps are *not* cancer but all should be professionally evaluated. A caffeine-free diet may decrease breast lumpiness, and a low-fat, high-fiber eating plan with little or no alcohol may reduce the risk of breast cancer. Suggestions for these changes are given in Chapter 15. If a cancer *is* found it is important to consider all the options for treatment. Consult with a surgeon or cancer specialist who keeps up with medical research, and find out about new surgical techniques that remove only part of the breast if the cancer is still small. Several helpful books on breast cancer are listed on page 186.

11

After carefully considering the pros and cons of hormone therapy, and consulting with her doctor, each woman must make a personal decision. Some will want to try estrogen to alleviate hot flashes, or may be advised by their doctors to use estrogen to prevent osteoporosis or premature menopause. Others will know immediately that they do not want to take ERT. Still others may have the health problems listed below that make it unwise for them to take ERT in any case.

Should You Take ERT? A Self-Rating Scale

Women with These Problems Should Avoid ERT:

Cancer of the breast or uterus

Heart disease, especially if chest pain is present

Serious high blood pressure

A history of blood clots in the veins or lungs

A history of stroke

Diabetes

Serious migraine headaches

Liver disease

Gallstones or gall bladder disease

Large uterine fibroids

In addition, women who smoke have a higher risk of heart and circulatory disease, and should not take ERT unless absolutely necessary.

You may want to consider the following rating system to help you clarify your choice.

The Decision to Use ERT:
A Personal Rating Scale

This rating scale is designed to help you clarify your thinking on whether to take ERT, based on your own needs and your personal and family medical history. If you have had your ovaries removed by surgery at any age, you should give a high priority to ERT because you lack those ovarian hormones that are secreted throughout life (see Chapter 3). If you are under 45 with premature menopause, you should generally take hormones until age 45 or 50; at that time you can reevaluate your use based on this scale.

Since the risk of cancer of the uterus from estrogen use is virtually eliminated if progestins are added (see Chapter 10), this risk is not listed as a factor in the scale.

How to use the scale: The advantages and disadvantages of taking ERT are listed. Each has been explained more fully earlier in the text, and is summarized in the pages which follow. Read over each summary section, and then assign a rating from 0 to + + + to each item on the scale, depending on its importance to you.

Show your rating scale findings to your doctor, so you can both determine the best course for you.

Advantages of ERT

Elimination of hot flashes. As discussed in Chapter 4, the use of estrogen tablets is very effective against hot flashes. However, hot flashes will return if estrogen is stopped. Slow reduction of dosage can lessen but not eliminate this problem. Alternative methods to deal with hot flashes are discussed in Chapter 4. Give yourself a rating of 0 to + + + depending on the importance of this symptom to you.

Advantages and Disadvantages of ERT — A Personal Rating Scale

Advantages

0	+	+ +	+ + +	Elimination of hot flashes
0	+	+ +	+ + +	Elimination of vaginal soreness
0	+	+ +	+ + +	Reduced risk of brittle bones
0	+	+ +	+ + +	Possible decreased heart disease
0	+	+ +	+ + +	Other personal advantages _____

Disadvantages

0	+	+ +	+ + +	Possible increased risk of heart disease or stroke
0	+	+ +	+ + +	Possible increased risk of breast cancer
0	+	+ +	+ + +	Increased risk of gallbladder disease
0	+	+ +	+ + +	Possible growth of uterine fibroids
0	+	+ +	+ + +	More medical visits and expense
0	+	+ +	+ + +	Monthly periods continue
0	+	+ +	+ + +	Other personal disadvantages _____

0 = not important

+ = a little important

+ + = quite important

+ + + = very important.

Remember to read the text before you assign the ratings.

Elimination of vaginal soreness. Estrogen is very effective in eliminating vaginal soreness due to penetration. However, minimal amounts of vaginal estrogen cream also do this, as discussed in Chapter 10. If vaginal soreness is the only symptom you want to treat, you can use very small amounts of cream twice weekly and not take estrogen pills. In this case give yourself a 0 rating. If you don't have pain with vaginal penetration, give yourself a 0 rating. On the other hand, if estrogen creams are not satisfactory and you are considering estrogen pills, rate this item with a 0 to + + + depending on its importance to you.

Reduced risk of brittle bones. As discussed in Chapter 7, estrogen reduces the risk of brittle bones (osteoporosis) and fractures. To help you decide on the importance of this problem to you, look again at the table on page 56. You should know that experts in the field of osteoporosis do not currently agree on the importance of all these factors. There is much more to be learned about what causes and prevents osteoporosis in different people. Therefore, the rating you give yourself based on this table will reflect an approximate idea of your risk, not a precise one.

Check any items that apply to you on this table. If you have two or more checks on the *Genetic or Medical Factors* list, you should consider yourself at risk of developing osteoporosis. If you have no checks on the *Lifestyle Factors* list your risk is lowered; but if you have one or more checks on this list your risk is increased—unless, of course, you decide to change your habits! If you are *thin,* especially if you are a *thin smoker,* your risk of osteoporosis with fractures is high. If you are Black, you can consider that you are more protected from osteoporosis than other women, but you should pay attention nonetheless to the factors on the table. Based on your study of this table, give yourself an overall rating for the advantage of estrogen in decreasing brittle bones. If you have made no checks on either list of the osteoporosis table, give yourself a 0 rating. If you have checked one or more risk factors, rate the importance of this item as + (a little important), + + (quite important), or + + + (very important). This item is a difficult one. Think it over and consult with your doctor or nurse practitioner if possible. Reread Chapter 7 for more clarification of the issues.

Possible decreased risk of heart disease. The effects of estrogen on the development of heart disease are not entirely known. Several studies show that low-dose post-menopausal estrogens protect against heart attacks. If your uterus has been removed, so that you can take estrogen without an added progestin, you may lower your risk of heart disease by taking ERT. Be sure your blood pressure is not high and does not rise with estrogen therapy.

If your uterus is not removed, you must take a progestin for 10 to 14 days of each month along with estrogen to prevent uterine cancer. This may change or reverse the protective effect of estrogen on heart disease, as explained in the previous chapter.

Consult your doctor about this question, as it is confusing, and hopefully new research findings will be forthcoming.

To rate this advantage of ERT do the following: If you have had a hysterectomy, give yourself a rating of 0 to + + +, depending on the importance to you of a decreased risk of heart disease, based on your personal and family history. If you have a uterus and must therefore use a progestin, give yourself a 0 rating on this item.

Other personal advantages. Rate the importance of any other advantages of estrogen therapy that you may be aware of. Some women find that it increases their sex drive, helps reduce forgetfulness, or improves their mood. Since these effects are individual, you may need to try estrogen to determine its effects on you. Give yourself a 0 to + + + rating on each factor that is important to you.

Disadvantages of ERT

Possible increased risk of heart disease or stroke. When a progestin is added to estrogen to protect against uterine cancer, it may increase the risk of heart disease or stroke. Progestins change the type of fats in the blood stream, and make it more likely that damage to blood vessels may ultimately occur. Women who have not had a hysterectomy must use a progestin at the end of each month of estrogen pills. Until more is known, those with pre-existing risks of heart disease should proceed with caution. Pre-existing risks include smoking, high blood pressure, elevated cholesterol, diabetes, significant obesity, inactivity, and a close family history of heart attack or stroke. Consult with your doctor about these questions. If you have had a hysterectomy (and thus need not use progestin), give yourself a 0 rating on this item. If your uterus is intact, rate the risk from 0 to + + +, depending on the importance of this factor to you.

Possible increased risk of breast cancer. The effects of ERT on the development of breast cancer are controversial. Several studies have shown a small increased risk after long-term hormone use, while other studies have not shown this association. Until more is known, women with a higher risk of breast cancer based on family history, their not having borne children, or their having a prior breast biopsy showing "atypical proliferation," should proceed with caution. Consult with your doctor about your risk in this area.

Give yourself a rating of 0 to + + + based on your personal appraisal of these factors.

Increased risk of gallbladder disease. Gallstones, gallbladder pain, and the necessity for surgical removal of the gallbladder have occurred with greater frequency with estrogen use in several studies. Women most at risk for gallstones are those who are obese, have high cholesterol levels in the blood, or have diabetes, Crohn's disease, or some other rare illnesses. Native American women from the Southwest frequently develop gallstones. A high fiber diet protects against gallbladder disease.

Give yourself a rating of 0 to + + + based on your appraisal of your risks.

Possible growth of uterine fibroids. Estrogen can cause uterine fibroid tumors to grow larger. While these benign tumors usually shrink after the menopause, they can remain large or continue to grow when ERT is taken. If you do not have fibroids, you can give this item a 0 rating. If your doctor has told you that you have fibroids of any significant size, discuss this question with her or him, and give yourself a rating between + and + + +.

More medical visits and expenses. Women who use post-menopausal hormones need checkups every 6 to 12 months. They will need more laboratory tests, and will spend money every month buying medications. Give yourself a rating of 0 to + + + based on your feelings about this.

Monthly periods continue. When estrogen with an added progestin is taken after the menopause, a monthly flow continues, necessitating the use of pads or tampons. This flow rarely causes serious cramps.

Give yourself a rating from 0 to + + + depending on your feelings about this. Some women may welcome this menstrual flow and put the score in the advantage column.

Other personal disadvantages. Rate the importance to you of any other disadvantage of estrogen therapy that applies to you. Some women find it difficult to remember to take daily pills, do not like the way they feel on ERT, or think that such a use of hormones is against nature's plan for their bodies. Rate your personal appraisal of these disadvantages from 0 to + + +.

When you have rated each item on the table of Advantages and Disadvantages of ERT (page 105) look at the table for some time and think about it. You need not compare your total score for advantages and disadvantages. The table is not designed to give you a numerical score, but to summarize the data and let you judge how strongly you feel about the benefits and risks of ERT as they are currently known.

Be sure to discuss your questions and conclusions with your doctor or nurse practitioner, both now and as your knowledge increases and your feelings change. Remember that many women have tried estrogen and then stopped it — your decision does not have to be final. Remember also the alternative treatments for menopausal problems discussed in this book.

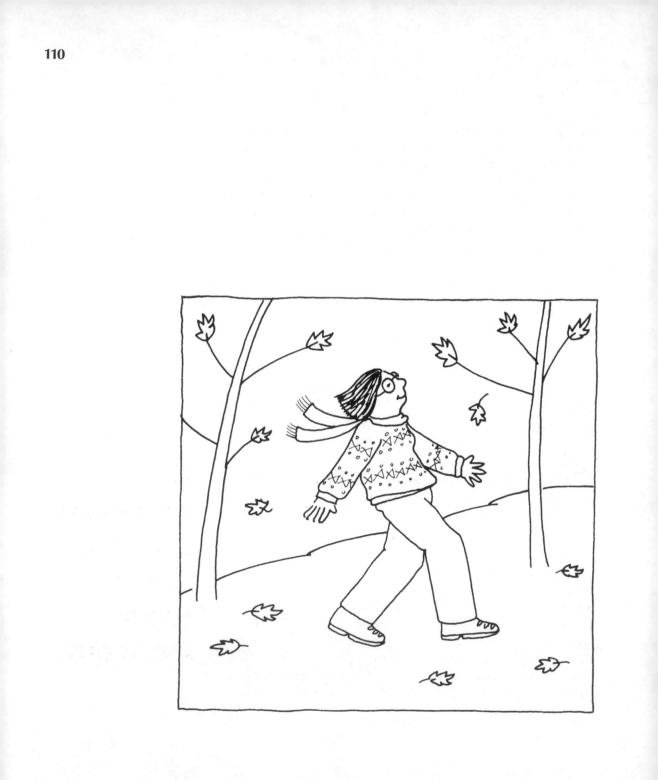

I'm not exactly sure what lies ahead for me . . . this new young woman. It's a brand new role for me. All this freedom to be myself at long last. To really be myself. Not what someone said I should be . . . not what someone expected me to be. I don't know what is around the bend . . . but I do know that I'm on the path that takes me there . . . my feet are willing and light . . . my spirit is free . . . and I am feeling . . . wonderful.

— Gloria, age 50, after her menopause

As menstrual periods stop, women enter a time in their lives which can be vital and new. Margaret Mead, the well-known anthropologist with an interest in women's roles, coined the term "post-menopausal zest" for this period.

What is this state? Zest is a quality that gives our lives relish, stimulation, and keen enjoyment. How do we find and keep a sense of zest for living in mid-life? Everyone knows some older people who have it — who are vital and involved in the world around them. We also know people of the same age who are depressed, ailing, or reclusive. In this section we will consider ways to find and keep a zestful outlook in the second half of life. Some of these concepts have been touched on earlier in this book in relation to special problems of the menopause; but most ways to keep zestful are as useful to men as to women.

POST-MENOPAUSAL ZEST (PMZ)... HOW TO FIND IT AND KEEP IT

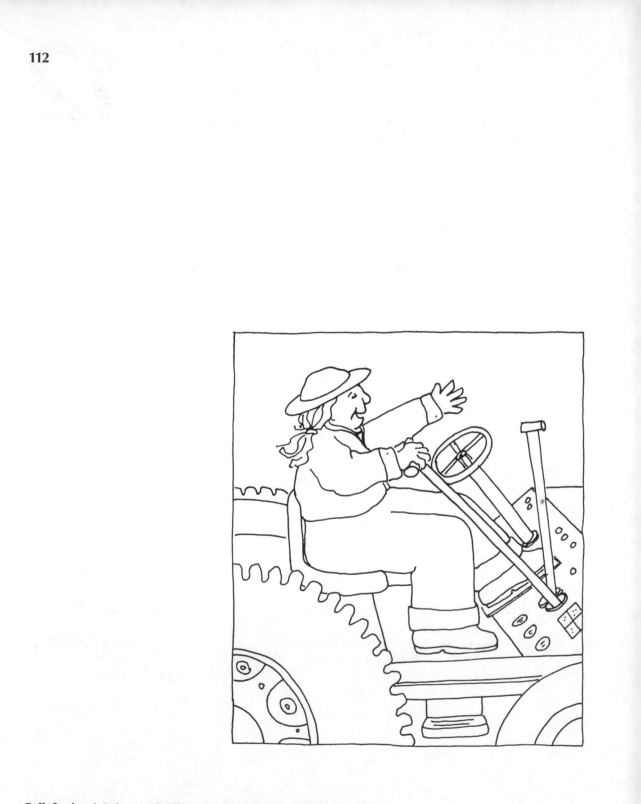

Beliefs about Aging: Unfolding and Growing, or Dying on the Vine?

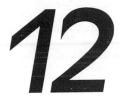

The greatest discovery of any generation is that human beings can alter their lives by altering their attitudes of mind.
— *Albert Schweitzer*

Aging is the term for a continuous process of growth through life.
— *Maggie Kuhn*

*J*anet was very involved in running her farm, and at 55 she was attending extension courses at night to learn more about new methods of managing pests with fewer chemicals. Her husband had died of a sudden heart attack when she was 48. Both her daughters had gone to the state capital to work. At first she was overwhelmed and thought of selling the farm, but gradually she began to see that she could handle it herself with some new techniques, different cash crops, and the help of a young couple who came to live with her. She realized that she came from a long line of strong farm women who had overcome great hardships in coming to this country and living off the land. She enjoyed the challenges of outdoor work and farm management, and found she could do many things she previously left to her husband. When people admired her work she was fond of saying, "These past years have sure taught this old dog some new tricks."

Beliefs about Aging: Unfolding and Growing, or Dying on the Vine?

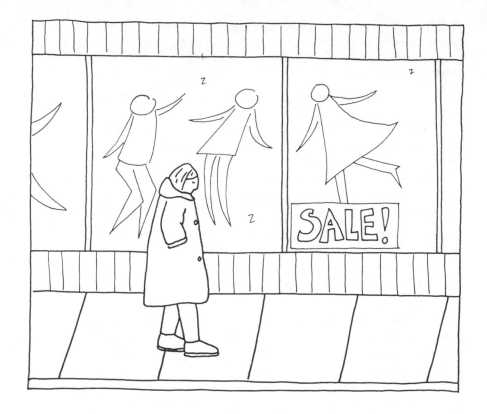

Rebecca lost her job as a secretary after 20 years when the firm went bankrupt. She was 52, and lived alone. She managed to find occasional jobs in a temporary agency but felt financially and emotionally insecure. She called her son on the phone daily and wanted to move in with him, but he had a wife and small child and did not welcome the idea, although he did send her some money every month. Rebecca increased her daily dose of estrogen and took antidepressants, but she still felt terrible. She saw no future for herself. She felt she had alienated most of her old friends by refusing to go out with them or crying so easily. At the mental health clinic they suggested she be hospitalized and consider shock treatments, but she had no insurance and was frightened by this idea. Rebecca remained depressed, often contemplating suicide but being restrained by her religious beliefs and her attachment to her son and grandchild. After a few years, she slowly began to improve. A friend gave her some back copies of Prevention magazine, and she started taking vitamins and eating healthier food. She felt a little better, but still had trouble seeing herself as valuable or

important in any way. Besides her son and her part-time jobs, she had very few connections to the world around her. She didn't see how she could possibly start any new activities or get any new interests at this stage in her life.

We are subtly but profoundly influenced by the beliefs our culture holds about aging. Often our view of other women or ourselves in the menopausal years is a composite of how we saw our own mothers and other family members, and what we glean from the media. Many women have negative memories of their own mothers' menopausal symptoms and a strong dread of aging. Others have positive, powerful, or serene role models in their families.

It is worth spending some time understanding what your own inner views of the menopause and aging may be. Close your eyes and picture a woman of 50, in her menopausal years. What does she look like, how does she feel, how does she move and speak? Write down three adjectives to describe this woman. Do the same for a woman of 60, and then one of 70. Visualize them in your imagination, and then describe each with three adjectives. Look over what you have written, and get an idea of your own fantasies and beliefs about aging. Do you like these women? Do you want to be like them as you age? If not, what do you want to be like when you are 50, 60, and 70?

Play the game again, and visualize *yourself* at each of those ages. Write down three adjectives to describe yourself at 50, 60, and 70 the way you really want to be. Now look at your two lists. Is your second list — with your personal ideals — different from your first list? What this exercise can do is show you that you don't have to be like your imaginary pictures of an older woman if you don't want to be. You can be your unique self, growing older in your own fashion.

Although our culture may have a stereotyped view of men and women at various ages, projected in television, movies, and advertisements, real people are incredibly diverse. We are usually happier if we value our uniqueness and do not try to make our-selves over to fit the cultural mold. Women who do not accept the prevalent belief that their worth as females depends on youthful sex appeal can value wisdom and strength in middle age. However, if you listen to messages like, "You can't teach an old dog new tricks"—you can't learn a new skill, sport, language, or instrument after age 15 or 25 or some other cutoff date—you will make these prophecies come true for yourself.

To break away from negative belief systems, it helps to find friends who are excited about life after 50 and talk to them about their outlooks, activities, and plans. Find out about organizations like the Gray Panthers, composed of people of all ages who want to change society and combat ageism. Gradually you will see a more positive view of human potential in aging which you can incorporate into your consciousness. Let your fantasy and imagination dwell on these new role models instead of the negative stereotypes the media offer. Instead of a nagging wife in curlers, think of Margaret Mead, Golda Meir, or Maggie Kuhn, founder of the Gray Panthers. Why not?

Stay Connected to the World Around You

Numerous studies of aging have shown that people connected to a network of others are happier and live longer. While spending time alone is important for quiet self-renewal and creativity, it can be a problem for depressed people who spend it watching television or drinking. Connections to the natural world are also important—animals, plants, walks in the park, and hikes in nature. These activities keep us aware of the web of life and help to combat depression.

Community and political involvement are important tasks for the second half of life. We need to use our experience to help direct the larger society in which we live, in whatever way seems most appropriate. Voting is important, but many people can give more than a vote to a cause or organization they believe in. Such individual efforts are the lifeblood of our democratic society, and can give great meaning to those who participate in them.

Middle-aged people who believe in their abilities to keep on learning and giving are doing many things in our society. They are returning to college, sometimes finishing a degree at 60 or 70 that they couldn't pursue in their 20s. They are involved in

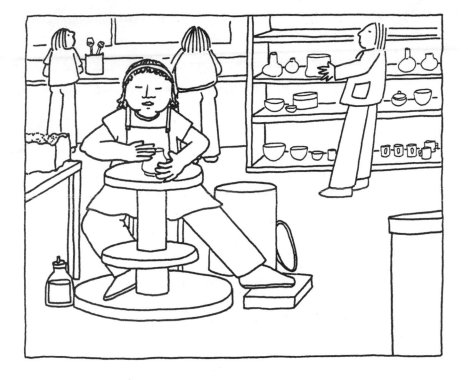

community affairs, politics, or crafts, in addition to holding
down jobs. Sometimes they are finding new ways to earn income
from their interests. Women who have been mothers, in particular, must redefine themselves in mid-life when the parent role has
ended. This is important as a bridge to the future, to keep life vital
into old age.

One of our important life jobs is to keep discovering and
growing until we die. As one sage woman puts it, we must
uncover our inner design. This means discovering who we
are — amid or beyond our many roles as worker, parent, spouse,
or lover — and what really gives our lives meaning. What excites
us and makes us grow? What can we best give to the world
around us? Such answers are obvious to some people but hard for
others to find. Answers vary at different times in our lives.
Getting even a partial answer to these questions is energizing.
Knowing where you are going in life is an important part of
post-menopausal zest.

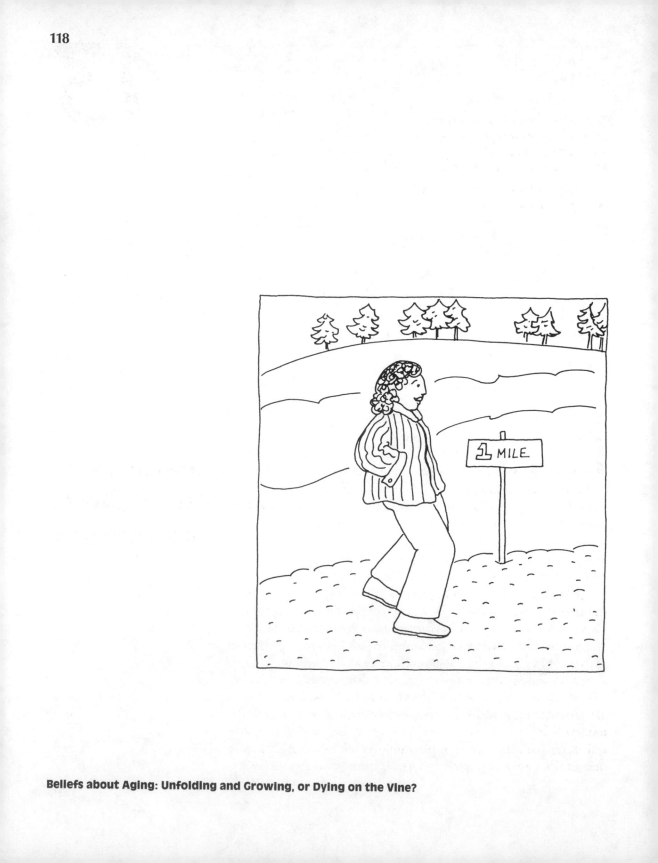

Beliefs about Aging: Unfolding and Growing, or Dying on the Vine?

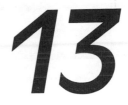

The softest thing in the universe
Overcomes the hardest thing in the universe.
That without substance can enter where there is no room.
Hence I know the value of non-action.

Teaching without words and work without doing
Are understood by very few.

— *Lao Tsu*

Relaxation: Calming Down and Letting Go

*L*ife is constantly challenging, both physically and psychologically — and cannot be otherwise. Our innate urges to survive, relate to others, learn, and master our environment cause change and conflict. The idea that life can be lived without stress, or that happiness is found in perpetual relaxation is a common misinterpretation of the aims of stress-reduction techniques. It has been aptly named "the Elysian Fields fallacy."

What we need is the ability to alternate between being alert and energetic on the one hand, and relaxed and calm on the other. This sounds obvious, but many people have difficulty letting go of the tension they accumulate during the day. They are perpetually switched "on" and can only turn themselves "off" with alcohol, tranquilizers, or exhaustion and fitful sleep. Some of the reasons for this are obvious. Urban living is crowded, noisy, mechanized, and rushed. The media bombards people with sounds of urgency and scenes of violence or disaster. Competition and "hurry sickness" are an important part of our culture. "Hurry sickness" is a term discussed by Drs. Friedman and Rosenman in

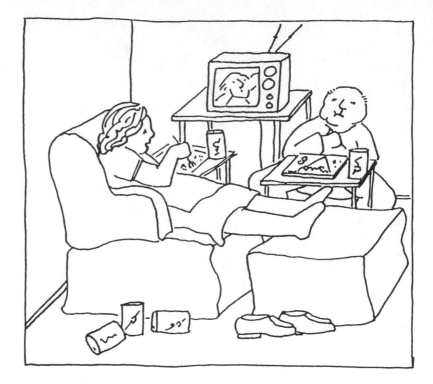

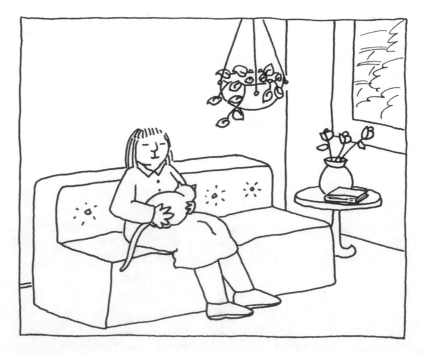

Relaxation: Calming Down and Letting Go

their book *Type A Behavior and Your Heart;* it refers to pervasive feelings of urgency and time pressure which may contribute to heart disease and other common illnesses of contemporary life.

It is overly simplistic to say that heart disease, cancer, allergies, or ulcers are "caused" by excessive stress alone. There are many other genetic, environmental, and lifestyle factors involved in these illnesses. However, we can say that many illnesses are aggravated by prolonged, excessive tension — whether it stems from noise, rush, and overwork, or from fear, anger, and self-blame. Conversely, sick people often recover faster, with less pain and disability, when they learn to get rid of excessive tension. Animal research shows that stress or fear depress the immune system, making the body more vulnerable to infectious agents or cancer.

Let's consider some of the factors in everyday life which can be changed to lower tension and restore balance to our nervous systems.

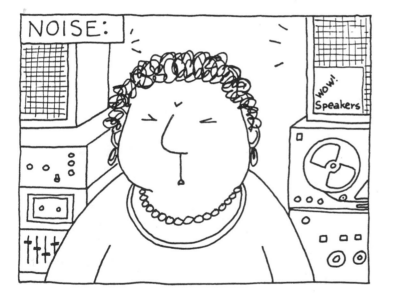

Noise is an obvious place to start. Many people are constantly bombarded by noise, which causes tension, fatigue, and blood pressure elevation. Noise at work and in cities may be unavoidable, but noise at home can be minimized. Anyone who feels

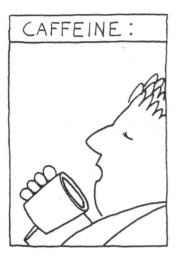

CAFFEINE:

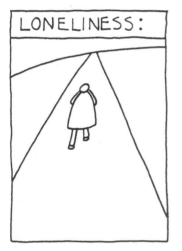

LONELINESS:

overstressed should experiment with turning off the television, radio, and loud music, and living with silence. Even short periods of silence during the day are helpful to enable our nervous systems to rebalance. In Quaker tradition, silence is used for worship and for the beginning and end of business meetings and ceremonies. It enables the participants to renew themselves, hear their inner spirits, and go forth to be effective in dealing with the problems of the world.

Many people repeatedly drink coffee, tea, or colas during the day, giving themselves a caffeine high that comes from stimulation of the adrenal glands and the central nervous system. It is more difficult to relax under the influence of a stimulant drug. When people cut down on caffeine consumption or eliminate it completely, the results are striking. They frequently feel less stressed. They learn to identify when they are really tired and need to rest or relax. Moreover, they can relax more easily without needing a drink.

Both caffeine and alcohol can be pleasurable and useful drugs, but they are both physically addictive. We can be energized or relaxed without them and experience a quicker return to a natural state of being.

Loneliness and social isolation can be stressful. While many people need to spend time alone in order to relax or get in touch with their inner resources, most people need and enjoy a network of supportive friends and family. Working too hard, being too competitive, or moving too frequently makes it hard to maintain a circle of close friends. Recent research indicates that people with close-knit ties to family, friends, or religious or other social groups have lower mortality rates from all diseases than people who are socially isolated. It has been postulated in this regard that one reason women live longer than men may be related to their greater interest in social and family ties. Men and women who have the personality pattern that has been connected with heart attacks — competitive, hurried, impatient, and striving — may be more vulnerable because they cannot make good connections with other people.

Overwork is another common cause of excess tension. It is clear that hard work is necessary for survival, especially in times of economic difficulty. Change and technological progress make it hard to keep up in any field without constant efforts to learn new things and alter our belief systems. However, each person must assess whether she or he is taking on so much that constant feelings of rushing or incompleteness result. If there is literally no time in your day to relax, eat an unhurried meal, or talk with friends, your life plan may need reassessment. Quakers consider it important to limit one's work life to have enough time for family, friends, and activities connected to the Meeting. One well-known cancer specialist insists that his patients spend an hour a day doing something that involves play and fun. Norman Cousins has advocated "laugh therapy." It's better not to wait until you're seriously ill to follow these prescriptions!

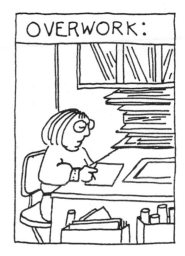

Inner tensions can be as destructive as those generated by the outside world. Anxiety, fear, grief, anger, self-blame, and poor self-image are words describing complex and unpleasant feelings that assault us and cause distress. Counseling with a trained psychotherapist is often an effective approach to these problems. In addition, many people have found the consistent use of relaxation techniques very helpful.

Relaxation Techniques

The goal of relaxation techniques is to enable people to return to a calm center after periods of activity. We understand intuitively that noise, conflict, anxiety, and hard work activate a part of our nervous system that is prepared for action in the struggle for survival. Another part of our nervous system functions when we feel peaceful, quietly aware, receptive, and relaxed. This part enables us to digest our food, sleep soundly, enjoy sexuality, and obtain relief from muscular pain. Pulse rate and blood pressure decrease. The immune system works more efficiently to prevent or overcome disease when we are relaxed. Many creative thoughts and important insights occur during times of quiet.

Relaxation exercises help in two ways: first, to return to a state of calm after episodes of anger, fear, or intense action, instead of feeling residues of emotional turmoil all day; and, second, to maintain inner balance most of the time, even during great stress, by having a sure sense of one's center and meaning. This comes with time, practice, and self-knowledge.

Many methods of relaxation are helpful; different ones are suitable for various needs and people. Meditation, silent prayer, yoga breathing methods, biofeedback, using a relaxation tape, or lying quietly in a warm bath are all ways to relax. Herbert Benson describes a simple breathing technique in his popular book, *The Relaxation Response*. A professor of medicine at Harvard University, Benson distilled the essence of meditation techniques from many cultures and religions into his prescription. Basically, it is this: Sit quietly and comfortably with your spine straight and your eyes closed. Silently say the word "one" in your mind with every exhalation. Focus your mind on your breathing and the word "one." When other thoughts come to you, let go of them.

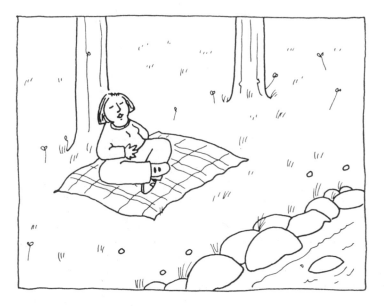

Develop a receptive and passive attitude. Do this for 10 minutes, twice a day. As you turn off the outside world with its noise and pressures, and turn away from your own thought processes, your body will enter a state of relaxation that has remarkable restorative effects.

I highly recommend *The Relaxation Response*. A perceptive reviewer said this book "can show those of us who are trapped in the Twentieth Century how to lower our blood pressures, change our harassed personalities, and, perhaps, even save our lives." To this I can add that many problems of middle age, including fear of aging and low self-esteem, are also helped by the relaxation response. People with certain illnesses, such as cancer, may want to use a relaxation technique that specifically relates to their problems. In this case, relaxation is combined with positive images of self-healing. The patient visualizes his or her immune system combatting and destroying the cancer. The use of such imagery to combat cancer is described by Carl and Stephanie Simonton in their book *Getting Well Again.* Simonton, a medical cancer specialist, advocates using their techniques *along with usual cancer treatments, not instead of them.* They have trained many counselors throughout the country in their imagery technique; a listing of counselors, tapes, and books can be obtained by writing:

Health Training and Research Center
P.O. Box 7237
Little Rock, AR 72217
Telephone: 501/224-1933

Carolyn, age 49, was a nonstop talker and a successful business-woman. She came to my office because of abdominal pain, digestive problems, and fatigue. She drank a lot of black coffee to keep her going at work, and smoked cigarettes to keep from overeating. She had written out a long list of physical symptoms that were troubling her, from headaches through back pain to cold feet. Almost none of her natural body functions were working smoothly. After listening to her problems and conducting a physical examination I suggested that we try a brief relaxation exercise as a model for what she could do at home. Carolyn found it very difficult to keep her eyes closed and not to talk for 5 minutes. "I couldn't wait to stop so I could tell you about another problem I have," she said. Then she laughed at herself and added, "I guess that's a part of my problem, isn't it?" Carolyn reluctantly embarked on some changes in the way she lived, including a 20-minute tub bath before dinner with the telephone unplugged, every night. In the year to follow she tried several relaxation techniques, and found that biofeedback worked best for her because she could measure her progress on the machine. She ultimately bought an inexpensive biofeedback machine to use at home. Most of her physical problems were resolved without drugs, and she slowly cut down on her coffee and cigarette use. She learned to be silent without feeling anxious, which made it easier for her to get along with other people.

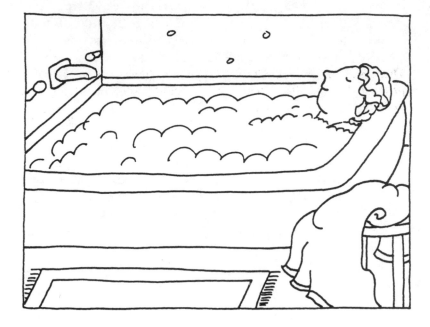

Relaxation: Calming Down and Letting Go

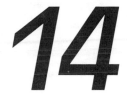

There is no drug in current or prospective use that holds as much promise for sustained health as a lifetime program of physical exercise.

— Dr. Walter Bortz

Use It or Lose It: Exercise in Mid-Life

O ur bodies are magnificently designed to move. But after a lifetime of sitting — in schools, offices, cars, and homes — we often end up pain-ridden and diseased. Doctors are slowly coming to understand that many of the changes we have attributed to aging are simply those that accompany physical inactivity. When young people stay in bed, they experience the same degenerative changes in heart and lungs, bones, muscles, body fat content, and digestive and nervous systems that we usually associate with growing old.

When middle-aged people exercise they can prevent, retard, or reverse many of these changes. The benefits of exercise include a reduced risk of heart disease and osteoporosis (brittle bones), easier weight control, improved appearance, decreased pain from many conditions, less depression, and better sleep. Let's examine these factors individually.

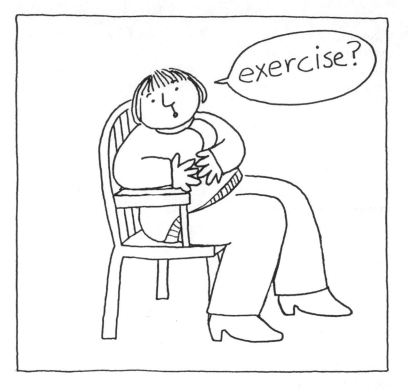

Heart Disease

Exercise helps prevent heart attacks. Though heart attack is the leading cause of death among women over 60, it is not inevitable. The kind of heart disease we have seen in this century is relatively new — arteries blocked by deposits of waxy cholesterol have never been seen with such frequency before. Our overconsumption of rich animal food, smoking, and physical inactivity seem to be the culprits. In past centuries, heart disease was mainly due to rheumatic fever and other infectious diseases, or birth defects, many of which can now be prevented or surgically remedied. Yet the only lasting hope for the new heart disease — cholesterol-plugged blood vessels — is lifestyle change. Surgery like the bypass, or replacement of blood vessels to the heart muscle, carry a surgical risk and only buy time. The vessels can become blocked again if the patient doesn't cut down on fat and start to exercise.

The combination of a low-fat, high-fiber diet and regular, vigorous exercise has a remarkable effect on the heart. Exercise makes the heart a more efficient pump, causing more blood circulation with each contraction and sending more oxygen to the muscles. As a result, you can do more without getting tired. This is what aerobic exercise is about. Any exercise is aerobic if it helps to condition the heart, lungs, and muscles to work more efficiently, or allows you to consume more oxygen during activity, and thereby experience less fatigue. If you start a brisk walking program, for example, you may feel tired after one or two miles at first. But a month of brisk walking conditions you so you can walk four or five miles with ease. Your heart will have been trained to become a better pump. It will beat more slowly when you are resting, because it will be stronger and send out more blood with each beat. It will have developed new blood vessels within the heart muscle to nourish itself with oxygen. Your chances of developing serious heart disease will have decreased. Equally important for the here and now, you will have developed more endurance and feel less fatigue throughout your daily activities. When you run for a bus, carry groceries upstairs, or folk dance, you will feel strong and capable rather than exhausted.

If you have exercised all your life, by all means continue daily during the menopause and beyond. If you have not exercised vigorously in the last month or two, begin with a walking program. Work up to three miles daily of brisk uninterrupted walking in comfortable, flat, walking shoes. Walking is an excellent form of aerobic exercise which you can continue for life with great benefit. So is swimming, or riding a stationary bicycle — a good alternative for stormy weather. As you start out with this program, check with a physician to assess the health of your heart and blood vessels. This is especially important if you have any history of heart disease, diabetes, high blood pressure, or chest pain. A doctor's checkup is very important for middle-aged people who have been inactive and plan to start jogging, aerobic dance, or competitive sports. It is safer to begin with a walking program and get conditioned gradually.

Readers interested in a full discussion of the benefits of exercise to the heart will enjoy the books of Kenneth Cooper, the cardiologist who started the worldwide enthusiasm for jogging. In *The Aerobics Way,* Cooper gives detailed charts for working up

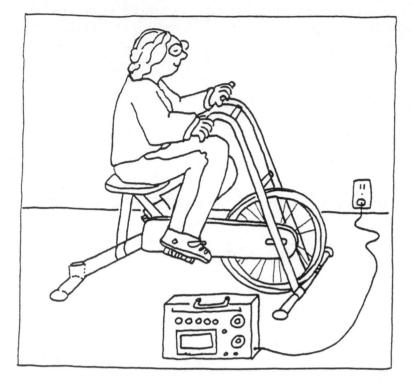

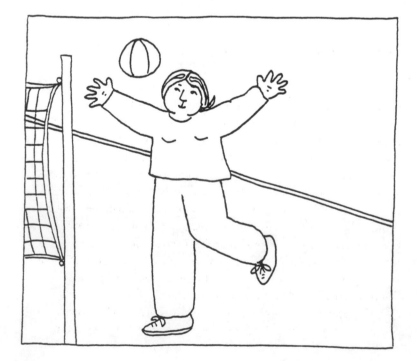

to optimal exercise times for each age group and each type of activity. For people ages 50 to 59, Dr. Cooper recommends working up to walking two and a half miles in thirty-seven minutes, four times per week, or riding a stationary bicycle twenty-five minutes, four times per week, with the controls (resistance) set so that a pulse rate of 150 is reached.

Similar prescriptions to be achieved gradually are given for jogging, jumping rope, swimming, stair-climbing, and other activities. Cooper's basic premise is that the heart becomes a more efficient muscular pump if you keep it trained. Just as our arm and leg muscles get stronger as we use them and weaker if we rest them, so does our heart muscle. A strong heart is a comforting companion in the second half of life.

But what about the waxy deposits of cholesterol in the blood vessels nourishing the heart? How does exercise prevent clogging these vessels? In several ways: It helps you burn calories rather than store them as fat. It encourages the formation of a larger network of blood vessels to nourish the heart muscle. In addition, it makes the blood less likely to clot by increasing natural anti-clotting factors. Conversely, inactivity makes clotting more likely. This is another reason why heart attacks and strokes are less likely if you exercise regularly.

Osteoporosis

The brittle bone problem of middle-aged and elderly women is helped by exercise. Recent studies show encouraging results in preventing and reversing osteoporosis when women take up a consistent exercise program. The subject of osteoporosis is thoroughly discussed in Chapter 7, and will be only briefly reviewed here. Bone fractures and back pain from compressed vertebra are both outgrowths of progressive loss of calcium from the bones, which occurs in women after the menopause. Black women appear to be more or less immune from this condition, perhaps because of their stronger bone structures. Latina women from Central America also have fewer fractures. About 25% of Asian, white, and brown-skinned women develop painful fractures from slight injury after the menopause. The most effective approach to osteoporosis is prevention, and exercise is one important factor. People who are inactive, or confined to their beds, quickly lose calcium from their bones. Conversely, people who use their limbs and muscles vigorously develop thicker, stronger bones. Middle-aged and elderly women need a daily walking program for their lower bodies and some exercise

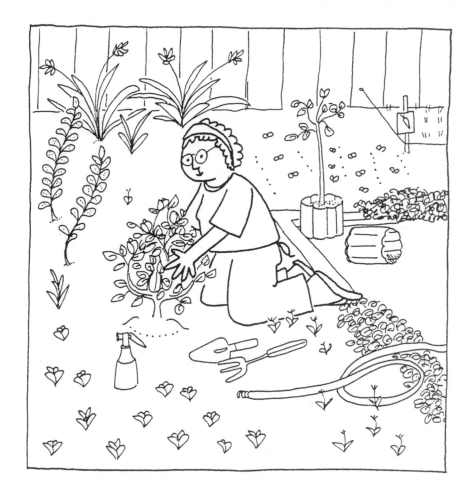

for their arms, like a racket sport, gardening, swimming, modified pushups, or lifting three- to five-pound dumbbells (or heavier ones, depending on their strength).

All movement helps — the thing to avoid is too much sitting or lying down. People with desk jobs should wear walking shoes to and from work and walk some of the way whenever possible. Use the stairs instead of the elevator for at least 5 stories. Do some walking during the lunch break. Jog in place or use a stationary bicycle at home, while listening to radio or watching television. However you do it, incorporate vigorous movement into your day, every day.

Even sick people and hospitalized patients should move around. Bones begin to lose calcium rapidly with bed rest. Enlightened doctors prescribe leg exercises to their postoperative patients and encourage them to start walking soon. If you spend the day at home ill, remember to move as well as to sleep. Get up every few hours, stretch, walk, and work your muscles gently. Your recovery will be easier, and your bones will stay strong.

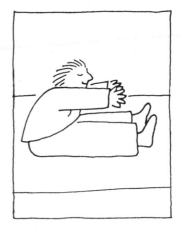

Weight Control

It's difficult to keep your weight in balance if you don't exercise. The small amount of food needed to sustain you in an inactive state keeps you chronically hungry and often undernourished. When small animals are kept in cages without an exercise wheel and given unlimited food, they tend to become obese. If they are given the opportunity to exercise along with unlimited food, they usually balance their intake with their energy output and maintain a normal weight. We function the same way. Weight loss is far easier if the dieter follows a daily program of walking, swimming, dance, or other movement.

In and after the menopause, women should not be too thin. The obsession with being slender in our society leads to great problems in self-image for most women at most ages. In the second half of life it is especially counterproductive, because thin women have less estrogen and greater problems with hot flashes, vaginal soreness, and osteoporosis (see Chapters 4, 5, and 7). This is not to say that real obesity is helpful; it has definite health risks also. Find the middle way for yourself—a weight that feels good and can be maintained.

Appearance

The person who works out with vigorous movement and stretching keeps a look of vitality and suppleness in the second half of life. A stiff body is not an inevitable part of aging. When middle-aged people start to exercise, amazing changes in their

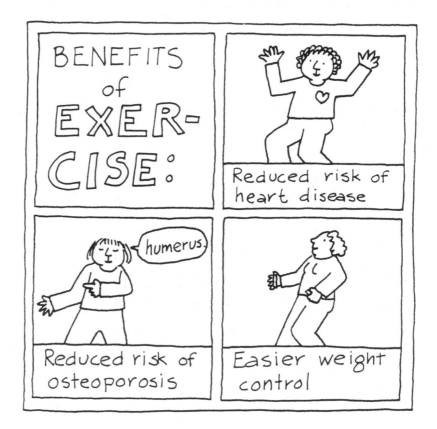

appearance are noticeable very quickly; a new grace comes from flexibility and energy. Yoga, dance, and Tai Chi are especially good forms of movement to impart youthful balance and grace throughout life.

Depression, Moods, and Sleep

Exercise has subtle but extremely beneficial effects on our moods. The physical, muscular activity of vigorous movement stimulates the brain, causing the release of substances which produce euphoria or "high" good feelings. Depression and physical pain are lessened. This is one reason why many joggers, dancers, or walkers get addicted to their activity. Some psychotherapists prescribe aerobic activity for depression and even go jogging with their patients. Any of us can experience a "natural high" through movement. Many people find they are able to give up tranquilizers or antidepressant drugs when they begin daily exercise. They sleep more soundly at night, even in the menopausal years when sleep is often troubled by hot flashes. Anyone with insomnia should try daily exercise as one form of treatment.

Stretching exercises also help to counteract emotional problems. Tension is always accompanied by physical muscular contraction. Chronically contracted muscles are tight and often sore. As we learn to stretch and relax our muscles, our minds become calmer. The amazing benefits of hatha yoga are related to this principle.

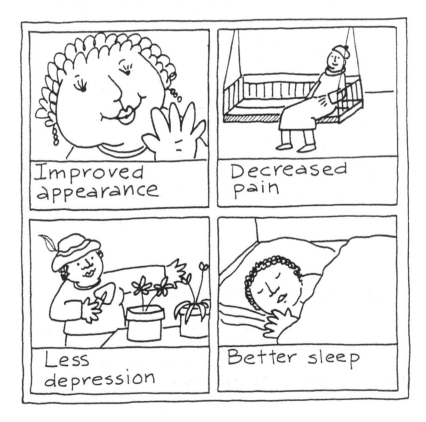

How to Start Exercising

The public has been exposed to lots of information about the benefits of exercise, and clearly it has made an impact. Joggers and aerobic dancers are all around us. Most adults, however, still lead fairly sedentary lives in our society, except for occasional weekend flings. The two most important realizations about exercise are these: First, you have to find activities you really enjoy or you won't keep them up; and second, you have to plan exercise into every day — just as you plan meals, shopping, and going to work. If you don't consciously make time for exercise you probably won't get it, especially if you live in a city. Even people whose work involves activity, such as waitresses, farmers, or gym teachers, often do not get both stretching and conditioning exercises at their work.

Finding an exercise activity that you really enjoy takes some introspection. Consider whether you want to take a class and be

---

Energetic Activity

    vigorous walking, hiking
    jogging, race walking
    vigorous dance, jazzercise, aerobics
    bicycling
    stationary bicycling
    jumping rope
    swimming
    racket sports
    energetic gardening or farm work
    sawing or splitting wood manually
    cross-country skiing

Stretching

    dance
    yoga
    many floor exercises

---

with people at a set time, or be by yourself at your own schedule. Do you want to exercise inside or out, with music or without it? Do you enjoy team sports and competition, or do you want individual exercise with your own thoughts and your own agenda? Was there anything you did in childhood that would really be fun to take up again, like swimming, jumping rope, biking, or dancing? Do you need different things on different days? Do you want to join a gym and work out on your lunch hour or after work, then have a sauna? Do you want to ride a stationary bike or use a rowing machine while you watch the news? Go over the table of energetic exercise and stretching, and think about those that seem right for you.

Remember to start slowly with any exercise if you have been inactive; patience and persistence really pay off. Above all, look at exercise as a way to put fun into your day, because the right kind for you will do just that.

Charlene was very unhappy about her body. At 53 she considered herself 40 pounds overweight, and she saw that she was gaining more each year. Yet she ate rather sparingly compared to many of her thinner friends, which seemed very unfair. Every piece of bread turned to fat on Charlene! She longed to go swimming at the community center pool, but felt much too embarrassed to show herself in a bathing suit. A friend urged her to join an exercise class, but for that she would have to wear a leotard! Even walking had gotten uncomfortable because of her weight. One day a belly dance teacher came to the community center to do a show. She was almost as fat as Charlene, but incredibly supple and sexual. Amazingly, she seemed happy with her body. Charlene thought about the dancer a great deal. She called a local studio that taught belly dancing and discussed it anonymously on the phone. The woman told her that belly dancers were proud of their bellies and that she should come try out a class. Charlene found she loved the music and the rhythmic hip swinging. She bought a tape and practiced daily at home or in class. Gradually she began to feel at home in her body again, for the first time in years. She became graceful and supple, and even lost a few inches and pounds. Many of her physical discomforts went away. Above all, she started to carry herself with pride.

Chapter *14*

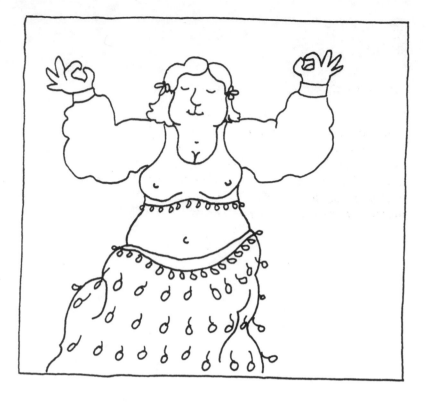

You are what you eat.

— *Anon.*

*And when you crush an apple with your teeth, say to it in
    your heart
"Your seeds shall live in my body,
And the buds of your tomorrow shall blossom in my heart,
And your fragrance shall be my breath,
And together we shall rejoice through all the seasons."*

— *Kahlil Gibran*

*E*ating the right food is an extremely important part of staying healthy and feeling connected to the natural world. The optimum diet for the menopause and middle age is high in vegetables, whole grains, fruit, and foods high in calcium. Such a diet can supply plenty of nutrients without causing obesity or heart disease. One advantage of this healthy diet is that it is delicious, another that it is less expensive than a diet centered around meat and canned or packaged foods. When people change to a better diet, they often notice that many health problems slowly disappear. Energy increases, weight stabilizes, hair gains luster and stops falling out, skin looks better, gums stop bleeding, and constipation disappears. Let's look at the individual elements of a healthy diet and understand their pros and cons. At the end of this chapter are some recipes and suggested menus.

Nutrition: All about Eating and Drinking

Whole grains

Grains are delicious and can be cooked in many ways: whole — as in brown rice; cracked or rolled — as in oatmeal; or ground into wholegrain flours. The grain family includes wheat, rye, triticale, rice, oats, barley, corn, millet, buckwheat (kasha), and wild rice. Although grains have been a staple food for most of recorded human history, they have recently acquired the reputation of being high in calories. Perhaps this is because of what we put on them: butter, cheese, gravy, and mayonnaise! A slice of whole grain bread has about 90 calories, a cup of cooked brown rice about 200 calories. Asian people, who live on a rice-based diet, are mainly slim, in contrast to Westerners on a meat(fat)-based diet. The fiber in whole grains helps you eat more slowly and fill up naturally, so you won't overeat. In general, it is the fat in our food that makes us fat, not the grains, potatoes, and vegetables.

The medical advantages of whole grains are worth thinking about. Everyone is aware that something called fiber is good for you and relieves constipation. Fiber, the indigestible part of plant foods, is found in different forms in grains, beans, vegetables, and fruits. People who eat a diet high in fiber have a lower risk of contracting cancer of the colon, and also have fewer problems with many gastrointestinal diseases, such as diverticulitis, hiatus hernia, and appendicitis. They also have lower cholesterol levels

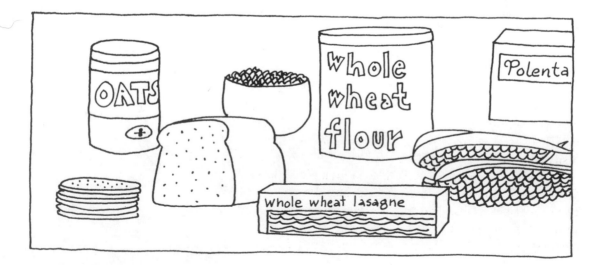

in the blood, even after eating the same amount of cholesterol in their food. This decreases their risk of heart attack.

It is also possible that a high-fiber, low-fat diet protects women against breast cancer. Women in Asia and Africa consume much less fat and three times more fiber than we do, and have a lower incidence of breast cancer than American women. Vegetarian women in the United States whose diet is lower in fat and higher in fiber, have less breast cancer than meat eaters. Many people add bran to their food in order to get more fiber. This is a good first step, but eating 100% whole grains makes more sense for your health. Bran is only one of the elements removed in making white flour or white rice. The germ of the wheat or rice kernel is the other part removed; it contains the B vitamins, vitamin E, and other nutrients.

Here are some guidelines for using whole grains. Buy or make your own whole grain bread without added white flour or sugars. Use brown rice, rolled oats (not the instant kind), rye crackers, fresh corn, corn tortillas, polenta, and buckwheat groats (kasha). Start the day with a whole grain cereal. Use whole wheat pasta, available at health food stores or food co-ops. Read a book like *The New Laurel's Kitchen* or the tenth anniversary edition of *Diet for a Small Planet* for easy ways to cook with these grains. Gradually shift away from white bread, cakes, donuts, and pastries to these healthier foods. If you like to bake desserts, use whole wheat pastry flour, which is entirely interchangeable with the white variety. Try plain popcorn for a snack.

Beans

Beans are excellent foods for several reasons. They are high in protein and low in fat. Any bean combined with any grain gives you protein of the same quality as meat, fish, eggs, or milk. For example, a serving of baked beans or split pea soup combined with rice, bread, or corn gives you protein as complete as that in meat. Vegetarians are well aware of this, and often find they can easily maintain their desired weight.

Another advantage of beans is their high fiber content. The fibrous cover around the bean slows its breakdown in the digestive process, so its nutrients are absorbed more slowly than other foods. Beans are considered the ideal food for people with diabetes because their slow regular absorption minimizes the need for

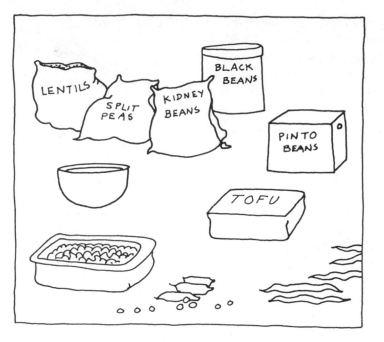

insulin. If you are bothered by intestinal gas when you eat beans, cover the dry beans with plenty of water and let them soak for 12 hours. Throw away the soaking water, rinse the beans, and then cook them in fresh water. This process eliminates certain starches that cause intestinal gas. Also, try fresh or frozen beans and peas, bean sprouts, and soybean foods like tofu and tempeh (found in oriental markets and natural food stores).

People who get much of their protein from beans and grains are helping the world food supply, as well as their own health. Sixteen pounds of grain and soybeans must be fed to beef cattle to produce one pound of meat. If more of us ate the grain and beans instead of the meat, huge amounts of agricultural land in this world could be planted with basic crops for the hungry. This idea is developed in *Diet for a Small Planet* and has caused many people to examine their usual ways of eating.

Vegetables

Vegetables have always been pushed by nutritionists and mothers because of their abundance of vitamins and minerals. Now we are learning more specifically that they may protect against cancer, infections, heart attacks, and stroke. The evidence comes from recent studies showing that people with high intakes of vitamin A from vegetables (yellow, orange, dark green, and red vegetables) have lower rates of certain cancers. Conversely, it has been found that people deficient in vitamin A may be more susceptible to cancer and infection because of an impaired immune system. These findings should not inspire the public to take large quantities of vitamin A in fish liver oil or capsules, since this fat-soluble form of vitamin A can be toxic in amounts above 20,000 IU daily. However, the water-soluble form of Vitamin A found in deeply colored vegetables and fruits is not toxic and can be eaten in large quantities. The vitamin C content of vegetables and fruits also plays a significant role in protection against disease, as do all the other abundant nutrients in these foods.

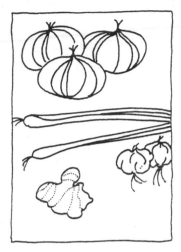

There is also evidence that vegetables in the cabbage family — cabbage, broccoli, Brussels sprouts, cauliflower, kale, and collards — protect against cancer by mechanisms not entirely understood at present.

The information that some vegetables protect from heart attack and stroke comes from studies on garlic and onions, which show that they lower levels of serum cholesterol and decrease the tendency of the blood to clot. Similar effects are seen with ginger root and certain mushrooms.

To obtain maximum nutrients from vegetables, they should be eaten raw in salads or lightly steamed. Water in which vegetables have been cooked should be kept and used as broth, because it is high in vitamins and minerals.

Sprouting is another way to obtain delicious food high in nutrients. As sprouts grow, their vitamin content increases,

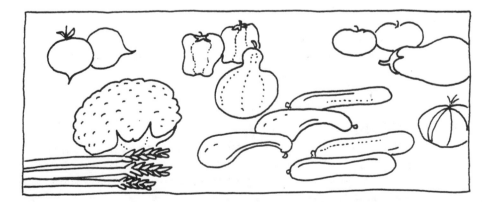

providing the benefits of fresh vegetables even in winter in northern areas. Anyone can make bean sprouts in the kitchen, from lentils, aduki beans, mung beans or many seeds. No other fresh crop is so easily obtained. Cover ¼ cup of small beans like lentils with water and soak in a glass jar for 12 to 24 hours. Rinse the beans and invert the jar after covering its mouth with cheesecloth or a fine meshed screen. Keep the jar inverted on your dish drying rack, rinsing the beans twice daily. The sprouts will be visible in a few days; eat them raw in salads or throw them into pasta or stir-fried vegetables at the end of cooking, so they stay crisp.

Potatoes and sweet potatoes are excellent foods which should not be avoided because of their alleged tendency to cause weight gain. They are not the problem — it is the oil, butter, and sour cream with which they are often prepared. Potatoes are best steamed or baked, and can be served with yogurt and chives or other seasonings. They are good sources of protein, vitamin C, and potassium, an important mineral for people with high blood pressure.

Sea vegetables are not used in Western cooking but are high in necessary trace minerals. With a little information, you can gather your own if you live on the coast; virtually all seaweed is edible. Easier still, you can buy small amounts of dried kelp and other sea vegetables at a natural foods or Oriental grocery store. Snip it into small pieces and add it to soup or stews. Books on Japanese, Philippine, or Hawaiian cooking give more details on the use of sea vegetables.

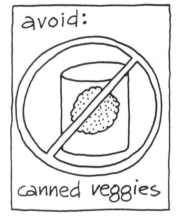

avoid: canned veggies

As far as possible, avoid canned or pickled vegetables, as their salt content is unusually high. Frozen vegetables are a better alternative when fresh produce is not available. Don't forget to make your own bean sprouts in the winter!

Fruits

Fruits are an excellent source of vitamins, minerals, and pleasure. Use them for snacks and desserts, instead of donuts, ice cream, or pastry. When friends and co-workers bring out cake, Valentine candy, or other sugary snacks, the conscientious eater can open a desk drawer, purse, or refrigerator and bring out fresh or dried fruit. For many people it is important to be supplied with healthy

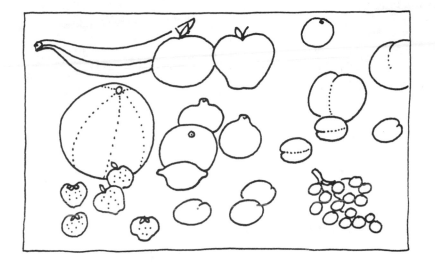

"reward" foods if they are to turn down the "treats" that lead to tooth decay and obesity.

It's true that fruits have a high sugar content, along with their vitamins and minerals. But their fiber content slows down the eating process and makes us full faster. In addition, the fiber of raw fruits has a stabilizing effect on blood sugar levels. If you eat two whole apples, your blood sugar will rise, just as it will if you drink the juice of those apples without their fibrous pulp. Two hours after the whole apple snack your blood sugar will be back to normal. However, two hours after the apple juice, your blood sugar will be significantly lower. This is because more insulin was released from your pancreas to help digest the quickly absorbed apple juice. The body responds to the juice alone in the same way it responds to simple sugar in soft drinks or desserts. The down-swing of blood sugar after the initial rise makes many people feel relatively shaky, and hungry soon again. The lesson here is — enjoy the whole fruit. Don't make a regular habit of drinking fruit juices.

Some people don't like fruit, are allergic to it, or are on diets that restrict it. They can get all the nutrients of fruits in vegetables. Others wonder how to avoid the pesticides sprayed on produce. Wash fruits and vegetables carefully before eating them. When possible, find a farmer's market where you can get locally grown produce, and look for stores that sell unsprayed or organic products. These markets and farmers deserve our support. One advantage of local produce is it has more nutrients because it is picked riper and stored only briefly. And finally, if you have a backyard or space for pots, start growing a few vegetables and fruits at home. The connection to the earth and the good eating are both nourishing.

Meat, poultry, and fish

All are tasty additions to a healthy diet in middle age, but none should be center stage. To have a low fat content in the diet, and thereby to decrease the risk of heart disease and cancers of the colon and breast, we should use meat as a flavoring for grains and vegetables rather than as the centerpiece of the meal. Oriental cooks do this by cutting up meat or fish and stir-frying it with onions, garlic, and vegetables. There are many other ways of changing to a low-fat, low-meat diet, such as making stews, casseroles, or soups using lean meat as a flavoring.

When cutting down on meat, it is not necessary to compensate with eggs and cheese; in fact, this defeats the purpose of achieving a lower fat content in the diet. Remember that a bean and whole grain combination provides high-quality protein — without added fat. You can eliminate meat entirely and be healthy! Vegetarians have good health records, with lower rates of heart disease and cancer than meat-eaters.

If you do like meat, how much is enough, and what kinds are best? Many heart specialists agree that middle-aged people should not eat more than one-quarter pound of lean meat daily. Trim all visible fat from red meat and choose the leanest cuts. Discard the skin of poultry. Don't use gravy. Avoid bacon, ham, lunch meat, and pressed or processed meats — they are high in fat, salt, and chemicals.

Frying or broiling meat at high temperatures develops certain cancer-causing products. Use a lower temperature for a longer time, or cover the meat and let it stew in its juices, staying at the boiling point.

Another reason to minimize flesh foods in mid-life is that they may contribute to osteoporosis, or brittle bones (see Chapter 7). There is evidence that high-protein diets cause a loss of calcium from the body. Several studies have shown that vegetarians have

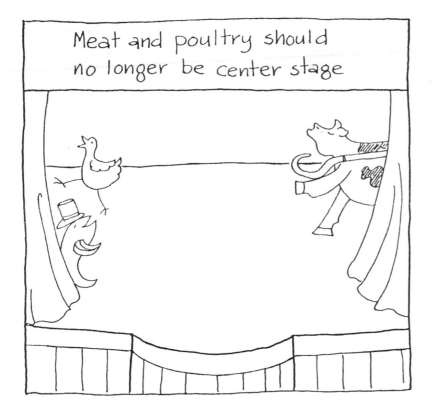

less osteoporosis than non-vegetarians. To prevent osteoporosis, it is better to get most of your animal protein from low-fat milk products.

Fish is the one flesh food that has a protective effect against heart disease, by virtue of the special kind of fat it contains. The oil in fish has been shown to lower blood levels of cholesterol and to counteract the tendency of blood to clot. People who eat large amounts of fish have strikingly lower rates of heart attack than meat eaters. Nutritionists are now suggesting that middle-aged men and women include fish in their diets two to three times per week, emphasizing the fatter fishes like salmon, mackerel, trout, and herring. If you eat canned fish, read the label carefully and drain any vegetable oil that is sometimes added. The mid-life woman interested in keeping her protein intake down could consider getting all her animal protein from fish and low-fat milk products instead of meat and poultry.

Milk, yogurt, and cheese

Nonfat and low-fat milk products are good foods for mid-life women because of their calcium content. Some adults lack the ability to digest milk sugar (lactose), and experience cramping, gas, and diarrhea after drinking milk. Sometimes such people can eat small servings of cultured milk such as yogurt, buttermilk, acidophilus milk, and kefir, where the milk sugar is partially digested already by the fermenting bacteria. Lact-Aid, a product sold in pharmacies, also predigests milk sugar and does so without making the milk sour. Soy "milk" can be used, especially in cooking, as a milk substitute.

Middle-aged people should avoid high-fat milk products such as butter, sour cream, ice cream, whipped cream, half-and-half, and large amounts of whole milk. About 75% of the calories in hard cheeses of all kinds are fat; hard cheeses should be used in small amounts for flavor. Low-fat cottage cheese (uncreamed), low-fat and nonfat yogurt, and nonfat milk are good choices, useful in cooking as well.

Many cultures do not use milk products and some Westerners avoid them because of digestive problems or dietary rules. Since calcium intake is so important in mid-life women, those who avoid milk should eat plenty of the other high-calcium foods listed in the following table, every day. Aim towards eating about

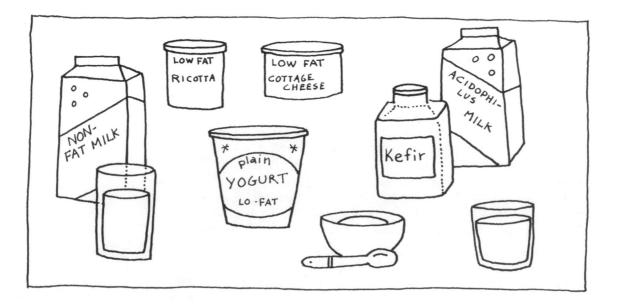

Food	Amount	Calcium Content
skim milk powder	¼ cup	400 mg
low-fat milk	1 cup	350 mg
yogurt	1 cup	300 mg
low-fat cottage cheese	1 cup	120 mg
collard greens, cooked	1 cup	360 mg
sardines, canned	8 medium	350 mg
blackstrap molasses	2 tablespoons	280 mg
sesame seed meal (tahini)	¼ cup	270 mg
kale, cooked	1 cup	200 mg
salmon, canned with bones	3 ounces	170 mg
broccoli, cooked	1 stalk	160 mg
tofu (soybean curd)	4 ounces	150 mg
corn tortillas	2	120 mg
calcium-fortified orange juice	1 cup	320 mg

Also — when making soup stock from bones, add one or two tablespoons of vinegar during the boiling process. The acid in the vinegar will dissolve the calcium out of the bones, providing a soup stock unusually rich in calcium.

300 mg of calcium at each meal from the foods listed in this or other nutrient tables. *The New Laurel's Kitchen* (Ten Speed Press, 1986) is an excellent vegetarian cookbook with useful tables of the calcium content in most foods.

Eggs

Eggs are a high-protein food many people enjoy; they're very useful in cooking. Because of the high cholesterol content of egg yolk, eggs have become controversial in recent years. Most cardiologists endorse the concept of a prudent diet where egg yolks are used in moderation — say three or four per week in middle age. It is much healthier to eat eggs poached, boiled, or baked in food than fried in fat. Cheese omelets or soufflés are very high in fat and cholesterol and should generally be avoided. Powdered or dried eggs in various packaged foods should be avoided, as there is evidence that processed, dried cholesterol

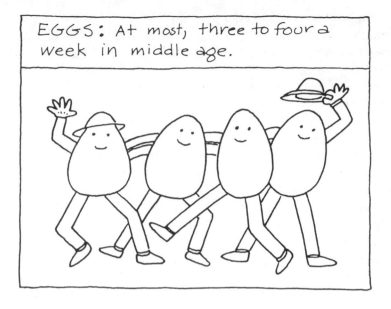

EGGS: At most, three to four a week in middle age.

may do more damage to blood vessels than the cholesterol in fresh food.

People who are limiting their fat and cholesterol intake often use egg white and avoid yolks completely. Farmers who raise their own chickens and eat their own eggs should know that chickens fed only grains and plant foods have about 50% less cholesterol in their eggs than chickens fed meat meal, fish meal, and poultry by-products.

Fat, Sugar, and Salt

Fats

Butter, margarine, oil, mayonnaise, cream, and lard are very high in calories, yet low in essential nutrients. Typical Americans consume about 40% of their calories in fat. This pattern of eating has been strongly linked to heart disease, stroke, and various cancers, especially cancer of the breast and colon. Recent evidence links a high-fat diet with high blood pressure, and change to a low-fat diet with rapid decrease in blood pressure. Since these diseases account for about half the deaths in the United States, it is important for our society to change our eating patterns, moving toward a much lower fat diet. Individuals can do this without major disruption if they do it thoughtfully.

For health, we do not need to add any fat or oil to our foods. Enough fat is obtained from whole grains, vegetables, and lean or low-fat animal products to satisfy our needs and allow us to absorb fat-soluble vitamins. Most people, however, want to have some fat in their diets for taste and a feeling of being full. Therefore, the key concept is to use fat sparingly. Use just a *little* butter, peanut butter, or hard cheese on your sandwich, with lots of vegetables and sprouts. Use just a *little* oil in frying and avoid deep-fried foods. (You can sauté food in broth or water instead of oil.) Make salad dressings with more lemon, vinegar, spices, and low-fat yogurt, and less oil or mayonnaise. Cut down by a third or more on the fat (butter, oil, egg yolk, and so on) required in recipes, and buy a low-fat cookbook.

For years nutritionists have advised the use of so-called polyunsaturated oils in cooking, such as safflower or corn oil, because these oils lower cholesterol levels in the blood. It has now been found that olive oil is the most effective and healthful oil of all in preventing heart disease. Olive oil is delicious in salads and can also be used for baking or to sauté foods. Use it sparingly, and in good health! The only drawback of olive oil is that it is more expensive than other oils.

Eat seeds and nuts sparingly, and be aware of their high fat content. Be very cautious with coconut or avocado. Think of these high-fat foods as flavorings, not the centerpiece of your meal or snack. Fill up on whole grains, vegetables, fruits, and some low-fat animal foods.

Most sweets, pastries, and dessert foods are high in fat. Read the labels carefully on all packaged foods, and avoid those with added fat and artificial ingredients. If you buy peanut butter, read the label and avoid varieties with hydrogenated oil. The hydrogenated (saturated) oil in peanut butter and many snack foods, as well as palm oil, palm kernel oil, coconut oil, and the fat in chocolate all raise your cholesterol count even though they contain no cholesterol themselves.

People who consciously change to a low-fat diet notice several pleasant differences. Many remark that they feel lighter, more energetic, and less sleepy after meals. They spend more time eating, and eat a greater volume of food, since low-fat foods are usually high in fiber and require more chewing. Yet they lose weight more easily and often stabilize at a weight considerably lower than before, without consciously dieting. Low-fat foods fill you up with fewer calories.

It's difficult, but not impossible, to find low-fat foods when you eat out. Much restaurant food is rich in butter, oil, cheese, and sauces. The conscientious eater can look for health-food restaurants and Japanese restaurants; fish or chicken without added butter, salad or baked potatoes with dressing on the side, and similar simple dishes. When making air travel reservations, ask for a vegetarian or low-cholesterol meal, or fresh fruit salad.

The recommendation to change to a low-fat diet is extremely important for staying well in the second half of life. It requires self-education and vigilance, but it's very rewarding in terms of one's energy and resistance to disease. It would be best to begin a low-fat diet in childhood, but middle age is not too late! The risk of heart disease increases after the menopause, and a very low-fat diet (plus exercise) is more important than ever.

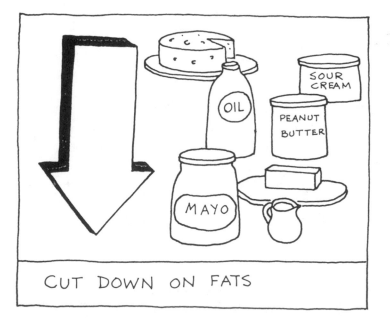

CUT DOWN ON FATS

Sugar

Simple white sucrose and its variations such as fructose are added to cakes, cookies, soft drinks, ice cream, candy, cold cereals, and many other packaged foods. Honey, maple sugar, and molasses are added to many health–food products. All these foods promote tooth decay and tooth loss, and represent substantial calories without nutrients. According to recent estimates, the average American eats 128 pounds of sugar per year! Sugar and syrups account for about one-fifth of our total calorie intake. When 40% of our calories come from fat and 20% from sugars, it's easy to see why many people in our society are overweight and prone to chronic illness.

For optimum health, eat sugary foods very sparingly, and satisfy sweet cravings with fresh and dried fruits. Many people do this by clearing all sugary foods out of their kitchens — from cookies to ice cream and soft drinks. They find they cannot avoid eating these foods if they are in the house. If you crave sweets, stock your kitchen with fruit, including prunes, raisins, dried figs, and dates. Take some to work, and reward yourself for saying "no" to morning donuts. The sugar you get in fruit is supplemented by vitamins, abundant potassium, and other minerals which aid in its digestion and in many body processes. Fruit has fiber but no added fat or salt. People who eat fruit but avoid refined sugar have far less tooth decay and other diseases of civilization.

Many people feel really addicted to sweet foods, in the sense that they crave ice cream, cookies, or chocolate daily and feel deprived without them. Usually these foods were associated with love and good times in childhood, and the association is hard to sever. It is best to work on this gradually, cutting down on sugary foods rather than cutting them out. Meanwhile, explore the beauty and bounty of whole natural foods and the exotic world of fruits. Focus your mind on the positive qualities of what you are gaining, not on what you are giving up.

Many people trying to lose weight use sugar substitutes such as aspartame and saccharin in desserts, soft drinks, and coffee. Saccharin is controversial because it causes bladder cancer in experimental animals. While this effect has not conclusively been shown in humans, the FDA requires a warning label about cancer on products with saccharin. Attempts to ban saccharin in the U.S. have been countered by great public pressure for its continued availability. Aspartame is a more recent sugar substitute which appears in diet soft drinks, packets for coffee and tea, and many diet desserts. Although it is intended to help with weight loss, aspartame has the paradoxical effect of increasing the desire to eat,

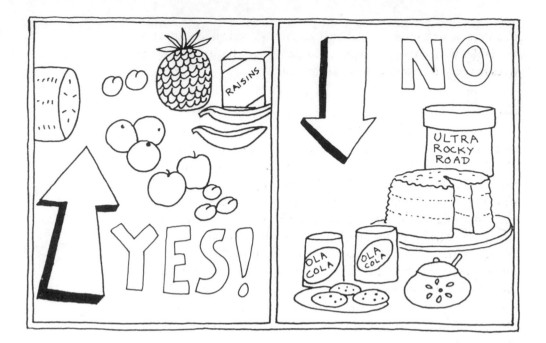

so that users of aspartame have *gained* significantly more weight than sugar users in a variety of careful studies! A number of neurologic side effects have been reported by people who habitually use aspartame in soft drinks and diet foods — dizziness, headache, insomnia, anxiety, panic attacks, and even seizures. If you eat artificial sweeteners, look carefully for side effects. Better still, satisfy your sweet tooth with an orange or a date.

In general, chemicals in food should be avoided. We already take in a considerable number of chemical substances from pesticides, herbicides, preservatives, and additives in food. It stands to reason that we should limit our intake of any chemical we don't need, especially if it is suspected of having adverse effects. In addition to avoiding artificial sweeteners, we should avoid artificial flavoring, coloring, and most other additives. Become a label reader and don't eat chemicals unless you know they are safe. The Center for Science in the Public Interest (CSPI, 1501 16th Street, NW, Washington, D.C. 20036) distributes a poster entitled *Chemical Cuisine* which lists safe and questionable preservatives and additives in food.

People who want a low-calorie alternative to diet soft drinks can drink low sodium mineral water mixed with a little fruit juice or a squeeze of lemon. Delicious low-salt vegetable juices are also available. With enough consumer demand, such healthful alternatives may soon be found in vending machines.

Salt

The sodium in table salt (sodium chloride), MSG (monosodium glutamate), and many packaged foods can contribute to high blood pressure and osteoporosis. Recent research has shown that the chloride part of sodium chloride may also raise blood pressure. For optimum health, most people should limit salt intake, and instead flavor food with onions, garlic, lemon juice, herbs, and spices. The body does require sodium, but usually we get enough of this element in vegetables, fruits, grains, and animal foods. In societies where little or no salt is added to food, there is virtually no problem with high blood pressure. Conversely, in societies like Japan, where food is highly salted, high blood pressure and stroke (a complication of high blood pressure) are very common.

From the perspective of good health, most food in the United States is oversalted. Not everyone develops severe blood pressure problems, but certain groups are more susceptible to it. Genetics plays a part here — people with family histories of high blood pressure are more likely to develop the problem if they salt their food. Blacks seem to be especially at risk for high blood pressure, and although this has been ascribed to increased stress from discrimination and pent-up rage, it may also be due to genetic susceptibility to salt intake.

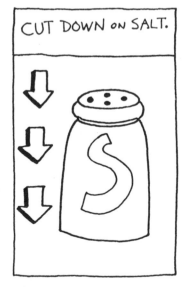

Limiting salt means cooking with little or no added salt and using herbs and other flavorings instead. It means avoiding much processed food, like canned soup, canned vegetables, pickles, olives, salted nuts, potato and tortilla chips, soy sauce, tamari, miso, and many packaged foods including packaged desserts. Any hard cheese should be used sparingly, because it is high in sodium as well as fat. Restaurant food is often overloaded with salt and monosodium glutamate, although some Oriental restaurants no longer use MSG or will omit it on request.

Clearly, it is difficult to be vigilant in this area. However, you can succeed in cutting down considerably and still enjoy food and life. In fact, a recent study of people who cut salt out of their diets because of high blood pressure revealed that they felt happier, less depressed, and less dependent on pain medications.

Salt is an acquired taste. Children brought up without it grow into adults who don't crave it. And adults can condition themselves gradually to enjoy food without added salt. People who have curtailed their salt intake are amazed at how salty ordinary American food tastes to them.

The drug treatment of high blood pressure often has undesirable side effects, such as fatigue, dizziness, or decreased sexual drive. There may also be unexpected long-term side effects to the powerful drugs now being used to combat hypertension. Though these drugs are necessary for some people, the medical profession is currently reevaluating their use. Many people can successfully bring down blood pressure without drugs by lowering their salt and fat intake, drinking very little alcohol, eating a diet high in vegetables, fruits, and calcium, exercising, and using relaxation techniques like yoga, meditation, and biofeedback.

Because of their high potassium content, fruits and vegetables are important in a program to reduce blood pressure. Potassium is an element similar to sodium, essential to life, but having the opposite effects on hypertension. Diets high in potassium and low in sodium tend to bring blood pressure down. Potassium is abundant in winter squashes, beans of all kinds, potatoes, leafy greens, and many fruits. When steaming or boiling vegetables, use the cooking water later as broth in order to retain all the potassium and other nutrients.

Convenience foods with minimum amounts of salt are available in the diet sections of large markets and in some health food stores. The government may soon require the labeling of foods according to their salt content. This simple measure has been advocated by the Center for Science in the Public Interest and other consumer medicine groups for many years. Such a requirement might create an immediate awareness among food-processing companies that they should provide lower salt products for health-conscious buyers.

Alcohol and Caffeine

Alcohol

Alcohol can produce pleasure, relaxation, sleep, relief from pain — and disease and death as well. The effects depend on the amount used and the metabolism and personality of the user. The menopausal woman, and middle-aged people in general, should treat it as a recreational drug to be used with care and respect. Our bodies cannot take as much abuse when we are 50 as when we were 20—hangovers last longer and feel worse! Let's examine the positive and negative effects of alcohol so we can make good decisions.

The positive aspects of alcohol for many people are that drinking enhances sociability, brings relaxation, and tastes and feels good. In addition, there is evidence that small amounts of alcohol increase a type of blood fat called HDL (high density lipoprotein) which protects against heart attack, and that in some societies moderate users of wine have lower heart disease mortality. (Exercise also increases HDL levels and protects against heart attacks.) Studies of people who live to age 90 or 100 have shown that many of them drink alcohol, usually in a social context with family and friends.

Positive remarks about alcohol must always be balanced with a recognition that this drug has also brought terrible personal tragedy and social disruption to our society. There are roughly 10 million alcoholics in the United States. Personality differences and biochemical individuality must explain why some people are addicted to heavy drinking, and why others feel toxic effects after small amounts.

There are several negative aspects of alcohol use in the menopause and beyond. Alcohol may act as a trigger for hot flashes. Heavy alcohol use has been associated with osteoporosis and fractures in older women for several reasons. Excess alcohol intake prevents bone cells from building new bone. Alcoholics often eat less calcium-rich food and excrete more calcium in their urine. They exercise less, and have more tendency to fall. Menopause may also be more troublesome because of the toxic effects of alcohol on the ovaries. In general, middle-aged women who have used large amounts of alcohol feel much better when they stop drinking. Nutrition improves when the empty calories of alcohol are replaced by healthy foods high in essential nutrients. Often many other health problems clear up—like excessive fatigue, joint and muscle pains, or hair, skin, and gum problems.

Several recent studies from the United States and Europe have shown an association between alcohol use and breast cancer. Relatively small amounts of alcohol, amounting to three drinks a week, were found to increase the risk of breast cancer by about

50%. A drink is defined as 5 ounces of wine, 12 ounces of beer, or an ounce of hard liquor. The increased risk was found to be stronger among women who were younger, leaner, and pre-menopausal, and was found regardless of whether or not the woman had other risk factors for breast cancer such as a family history of the disease or a late first birth. The conclusions drawn from these studies by the investigators at Harvard Medical School and the National Institutes of Health were that further research was needed to help clarify the possible mechanisms by which alcohol exerts this effect on the breasts. In the meantime, "the possibility that alcohol increases the risk of breast cancer should be considered in decisions about the use of alcoholic beverages." My advice to readers is to weigh these conclusions carefully and to consider switching to fruit juice and soda water on most occasions until more information is available.

Alcohol has been connected to high blood pressure when it is used in regular high doses. Anyone with a blood pressure problem would do well to drink only lightly, if at all.

Alcoholic beverages are made with many chemicals unknown to the consumer, since the federal government has consistently

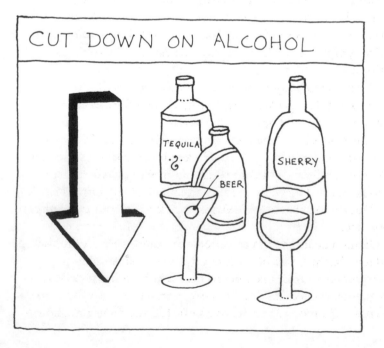

resisted enforcing labeling requirements for the wine, beer, and liquor industries. These chemicals may cause allergy, heart problems, or other illness in susceptible people. This is another reason to use alcohol with caution.

On the whole, it is best to be very careful with drinking in middle age. Analyze your drinking habits, and think about alternatives. Consider exercise, relaxation training, or counseling instead, if you feel you *must* drink daily to relax, enjoy dinner, or go to sleep. When you do drink, try not to exceed 5 ounces of wine, 12 ounces of beer, or 1½ ounces of hard liquor. If alcohol gives you heart palpitations (brandy and red wine can do this), or makes you dizzy or hung over, avoid it! Your body can't recuperate as easily in middle age, and must be treated with respect. Finally, if you have a compulsion to drink heavily or other problems with alcohol use, don't drink at all. Go to Alcoholics Anonymous instead.

Caffeine

Caffeine is a stimulant found in coffee, black and green tea, chocolate, many soft drinks, and some medicines. It affects the body in numerous ways, and is another recreational drug to be treated with caution. Most adults in our society use caffeine daily and are addicted to some degree to its stimulant properties. If deprived of caffeine, they may suffer mild to severe withdrawal symptoms, including fatigue, headache, irritability, and anxiety. These symptoms last from one to four days, and then leave entirely.

Many people enjoy the effects of caffeine, and like the taste of coffee or tea. Is this a safe drug in middle age? What are its pros and cons for the menopausal woman?

Caffeine is used because it decreases fatigue, and stimulates the mind and body to work faster. People think faster and often talk more under its influence. Caffeine enables people to concentrate harder and work longer at many mental and physical tasks. Meditation and states of relaxation are more difficult under the influence.

In high doses, however, caffeine can cause excessive tension and irritability. Users become edgy and uncomfortable, and overreact to stimuli. Their hearts beat faster; they may feel irregular extra beats as thumps in the chest. Blood pressure rises. Sleep is impaired, and a state of fatigue follows. This can make people use more caffeine and perpetuate the problem. All of these drug effects are more pronounced with aging.

Caffeine stimulates the smooth muscle of the gastrointestinal tract, causing some people to have diarrhea. Hence it should not be used at all by people with problems like inflammatory bowel disease (ulcerative colitis or Crohn's disease). Other people with chronic constipation use caffeine as a laxative. The same effect can be obtained, however, with a high-fiber diet of whole grains, beans, vegetables, and added bran.

Coffee has been associated with a rise in serum cholesterol, and thus may be implicated in heart disease.

Menopausal women frequently say caffeinated beverages increase hot flashes. This may be because caffeine speeds up metabolism and thereby increases body temperature. If hot flashes are a problem, cutting way down on caffeine can be very helpful.

Caffeine has been associated with the development of benign breast lumps in women. It appears to stimulate certain cellular growth factors in the breast, giving rise to more lumpiness and breast pain before periods. When women with breast lumps give up caffeine, the problem often regresses remarkably after four to six months. No relationship to breast cancer has been detected.

Very heavy coffee drinking (over 5 cups daily) has been related to calcium loss in women. It is apparently one factor that can lead to osteoporosis, especially if added to other risk factors (see Chapter 7).

In the menopause and in the second half of life, it is good to be tuned in to one's body messages. When you're tired, it is better to rest than to stimulate yourself artificially with a drug. Following the normal ebb and flow of the body's energies leads to a more peaceful and productive life.

For optimum health, it is best to cut down on caffeine consumption. Some people find they can easily do without it, and enjoy drinking herbal teas or cereal-based drinks like Postum or Cafix, that resemble coffee but are made from roasted grains. Others drink decaffeinated coffee; best are beans or instant coffee powder from which the caffeine is extracted by a process using hot water rather than chemical solvents. Still others use caffeine only when they really need the stimulation, rather than daily. If you use it, do so sparingly, and be aware of its effects on your system. Weak tea with milk is a safer stimulant than strong coffee.

Remember that cutting out caffeine may lead initially to a caffeine withdrawal state if you are a regular user. You may experience headache, lethargy, and irritability for a few days, but after this is over you will feel well again, and you will be free of a physiologic addiction.

Making Changes in Your Diet

A last thought on eating is that everyone makes changes according to his or her own timetable. Most people do better when changes are gradual, and when they emphasize the positive rather than feeling deprived. Women who are anxious about gaining weight may have an especially hard time changing from a diet that emphasizes animal protein, as they have been led to believe that other foods will make them fat. A gradual transition to a more plant-based diet is the key, with attention to your individual likes and dislikes. The menus and recipes in the following pages may give you some new ideas, and the bibliography at the end of this book lists helpful references on healthy eating.

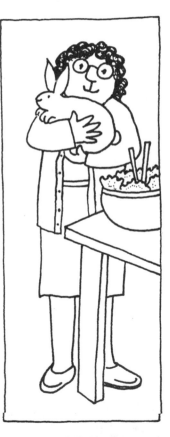

At 45, Lois had two experiences that shook her severely. Her brother had a serious heart attack, and she was operated on for a ruptured appendix. While recuperating in the hospital, Lois asked her doctor why she might have developed appendicitis. "Many people link this problem with a diet low in fiber," her doctor answered. "Appendicitis rarely occurs among people in Africa who eat large amounts of grains and vegetable foods." Lois thought of her own perpetual dieting on cottage cheese, hardboiled eggs, and meats — with occasional binges on cookies or ice cream. She found out while in the hospital that her serum cholesterol was 250, which worried her because of her brother's heart attack. Her doctor, who was very nutrition conscious, told her to bring her cholesterol value down below 180 to avoid the family pattern of heart disease. As she lay in bed, Lois realized a whole new way of eating was in order for her. She called a friend at work whom she had considered a health nut, and learned about the benefits of unfamiliar things like sprouted whole wheat bread, rolled oats, and pinto beans. Ultimately she found it easier to lose weight with this diet than it had been with her hardboiled eggs and meat. A year later her cholesterol level was well below 200, and Lois had become a health nut in her brother's eyes! She was trying to persuade him to try brown rice and salad instead of steak and french fries. "I draw the line at rabbit food," he would say. "Better to be a healthy rabbit than a man with a second heart attack," was Lois's answer.

Suggestions for healthy breakfast foods

Whole grain cereals

<u>Hot:</u> Oatmeal (not the instant kind)
Roman Meal
Wheatena
Zoom

<u>Cold:</u> Shredded wheat
Puffed wheat or rice
Grape Nuts
Uncle Sam
Any other cold cereal made without added sugars
or oil (read the label to be sure)

Milk products

Nonfat or low-fat milk
Nonfat or low-fat yogurt
Low-fat cottage cheese or part skim ricotta

Fruit

Oranges, apples, bananas, fresh fruits in season
Raisins and dates to sweeten cereal — instead of sugar
Unsweetened fruit spreads or mashed dates for toast
— instead of jam

Whole grain breads

Any bread made with 100% whole grain wheat flour
or mixed whole grain flours or sprouts
Whole grain English muffins
Whole grain pancakes or waffles
Corn tortillas — heat briefly and fill with beans, egg,
tofu, or cottage cheese

Tofu (bean curd)

Eat steamed, scrambled, or grilled; with onions,
curry, soy sauce, or other flavorings

Eggs

Boiled or poached (restrict yolks to 3 per week)
Use egg white to make an omelette with chopped
vegetables

High in Calcium

1 c	nonfat milk	300 mg
	low-fat milk	350 mg
	yogurt	300 mg
1 c	calcium-fortified orange juice	320 mg
½ c	low-fat cottage cheese	60 mg
¼ lb	tofu (soybean curd)	150 mg
2	corn tortillas	120 mg
1	medium orange (not juice)	50 mg

Try to eat foods with at least
300 mg of calcium at breakfast

Suggestions for healthy lunch foods

(* indicates recipes which can be found on pp. 164–166)

Whole grain bread sandwiches

Add fillings such as tomato, onion, cucumber, sprouts,
 a thin slice of cheese, mashed tofu, sesame tahini,
 sardines, or canned salmon

Salad

Mix vegetables, beans, sprouts, low-fat yogurt, or
 low-fat cottage cheese

Fruit

Eat whole, or cut up fruits with plain
 low-fat yogurt or cottage cheese

Soup

*Lentil, split pea, or other bean with vegetables

Breads

Corn tortillas
Whole grain bread
Whole grain crackers without added shortening
 (e.g. Ry-Krisp, Wasa Crispbread, Finn Crisp, Kavli
 Flatbread, Siljans Knacke)

Any dinner food listed below

Suggestions for healthy snack foods

Fresh fruit

Popcorn (air popped, without added butter)

Whole grain crackers, made without added shortening
 (Ry-Krisp, Wasa Crispbread, Finn Crisp, Kavli
 Flatbread, Siljans Knacke)

Slices of raw vegetables (carrots, green peppers,
 zucchini, cucumbers, tomatoes, and other vegetables)
 with tofu or cottage cheese dip

Plain low-fat yogurt with fresh or dried fruit

High in Calcium

¼ lb	tofu (soybean curd)	150 mg
1 oz	hard cheese	200 mg
1 c	low-fat cottage cheese	120 mg
1 c	nonfat milk	300 mg
	low-fat milk	350 mg
	low-fat yogurt	300 mg
8	medium canned sardines	350 mg
3 oz	canned salmon with bones	170 mg
2	corn tortillas	120 mg

Try to eat foods with at least
300 mg of calcium at lunch

Chapter *15*

High in Calcium

¼ lb	tofu (soybean curd)	150 mg
1 oz	hard cheese	200 mg
1 c	low-fat cottage cheese	120 mg
1 c	nonfat milk	300 mg
	low-fat milk	350 mg
	low-fat yogurt	300 mg
8	medium canned sardines	350 mg
3 oz	canned salmon with bones	170 mg
2	corn tortillas	120 mg
1 c	cooked collard greens	360 mg
1 c	bok choy	230 mg
1 c	kale	210 mg
1 c	mustard greens	180 mg
1	stalk broccoli	160 mg

Try to eat foods with at least 300 mg of calcium at dinner

Suggestions for healthy dinner foods

(* indicates recipes which can be found on pp. 164–166)

Whole wheat spaghetti

with *tomato-eggplant-garlic sauce, and parmesan cheese or toasted cashews

A "comprehensive salad"

Lettuce, bean sprouts, onion, sliced (raw or cooked green, yellow, and red) vegetables, toasted sunflower seeds or cashews, cottage cheese, sardines or salmon, with a *low-fat salad dressing. Goes well with baked white or sweet potatoes.

*Brown rice and *stir-fried vegetables*

with tofu, meat, or fish

Soup

*Lentil, split pea or other bean soup

Dessert

A bowl of cut up fresh fruit topped with yogurt, dates, raisins, toasted sunflower seeds or almonds (a good alternative to ice cream or other sweetened desserts)

Recipe suggestions

Lentil, Split Pea, or Bean Soup

A crock pot or slow cooker is ideal for cooking bean soup. Start it at night and it is ready in the morning; start it in the morning and it is ready for dinner. Add two cups of water for each cup of beans.

If you cook beans in a regular pot on the stove, add 3 to 4 cups water per cup of beans, and make sure the beans are always covered with water. Keep the pot partially covered — if covered tightly, it may boil over. Follow the directions on page 142 to prepare beans that do not give you intestinal gas.

Lentils and split peas cook in 1 to 1½ hours; larger beans take 3 to 4 hours.

Add seasonings such as garlic, onion, vegetables, herbs, or lemon juice in the last half-hour of cooking.

You can add significant calcium content to your soups by cooking them with a stock made from bones or egg shells. Boil bones of meat, poultry, or fish; for every quart of water add one tablespoon of vinegar. Simmer the stock for 3 to 4 hours. Remove the bones and refrigerate the stock overnight. Remove the fat that has hardened, and use the stock or freeze it for future use.

Vegetarians can simmer eggshells in water with added vinegar for one hour. Wrap them in cheesecloth, or strain broth before using.

Adding vinegar causes calcium to dissolve out of the bones or eggshells and enter the stock. The result is a low-fat calcium broth for people who don't like or cannot use milk products.

Low-Fat Salad Dressings and Dips

Make your own salad dressings with infinite variations in a blender. The basic ingredient is one cup of low-fat yogurt, buttermilk, or cottage cheese. Add a few tablespoons of minced onion, a garlic clove, dill weed, herbal seasonings, curry powder, or dry mustard. Add tomato juice for color and flavor. A table-spoon of olive oil adds richness (optional).

People who cannot use any milk products can get excellent results with tofu. Put ¼ pound of tofu in a blender, and add ¼ cup of tomato juice, one tablespoon of mild vinegar, one tablespoon of olive oil (optional), a dash of soy sauce or tamari, and season-ings such as garlic, onion, ginger, curry, or dill weed. Tofu tends to be bland; use more flavorings with it than you would with other bases.

Using less liquid will give you a tasty alternative to traditional party dips — and keep your guests wondering what it is!

For fruit salad, you can make a dressing of yogurt or tofu as a base, and add a banana or other fruit and a dash of cinnamon. Blend for a few seconds.

Tomato-Eggplant-Garlic Sauce

Using a heavy iron skillet or non-stick frying pan, sauté garlic slowly (as many cloves as you wish — the more the better!) in a small amount of olive oil (one tablespoon or less). Add seasonings such as basil, oregano, thyme, etc. Add a chopped eggplant, chopped fresh tomatoes or unsalted tomato sauce or tomato paste, mushrooms, green peas and other vegetables as desired, and enough water or broth to make the sauce simmer easily.

Cover and cook until the eggplant is thoroughly soft, about 20 to 30 minutes.

Serve over whole wheat pasta or brown rice.

Top with lightly toasted cashews or sunflower seeds (toast at 300 degrees for a few minutes) or grated parmesan cheese.

This recipe has many possible variations, depending on the ingredients on hand in your kitchen. It is an example of a low-fat vegetable sauce for pasta or rice. You can add crumbled tofu or cooked beans to increase the protein content. You can add chopped lean meat, fish, or poultry if desired, after the garlic and before the vegetables.

Stir-Fried Vegetable Dishes with Tofu, Meat, or Fish

Using a large heavy iron skillet or a non-stick frying pan, sauté two or three cloves of garlic (more if desired) in one tablespoon olive oil over low heat. Add chopped ginger root (one teaspoon or more) if desired. Add tofu cut into cubes, or chopped lean meat, poultry, or fish — about ¼ pound per person, and a little water, stock, or wine to allow the food to simmer and to prevent sticking. Stir frequently, keeping heat low.

After a few minutes, add chopped onion, mushrooms, and assorted chopped vegetables, starting with those which require the most cooking. Add a small amount of liquid, stir, and cover the pan for a minute or two between each addition. If bean sprouts are available, add them at the end, as you turn off the heat.

Serve over brown rice, bulgur wheat, kasha (buckwheat groats), or polenta (corn meal).

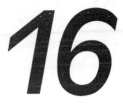

The most important practical problem confronting us in the nutritional field today is that of learning how to determine the specific nutritional needs of individuals. Typical individuals, as we have seen, have some needs for nutrients that are likely to be far from average.

— Dr. Roger Williams

Vitamins/ Minerals: Yes or No?

A health-conscious minority of the population takes vitamin and mineral supplements daily, with the view that their individual needs for certain nutrients may be larger than average, or their diets insufficient. Others consider supplements unnecessary, too troublesome, or too expensive. Nutrition experts often decry the inaccurate claims made for supplements, their potential toxicity in high doses, and the false sense of security they may impart to people whose diets are haphazard. With these viewpoints in mind, here's a simple regimen of supplements suitable for women in and after the menopause.

Calcium

Calcium is a mineral of great importance to the middle-aged woman, especially if she elects not to use estrogen replacement therapy. If a high-calcium diet is eaten throughout life and calcium

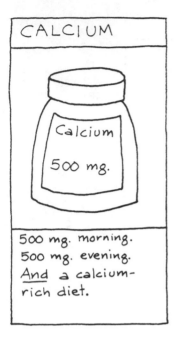

CALCIUM

Calcium

500 mg.

500 mg. morning.
500 mg. evening.
<u>And</u> a calcium-
rich diet.

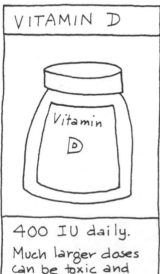

VITAMIN D

Vitamin

D

400 IU daily.
Much larger doses
can be toxic and
should be avoided.

supplements (500 mg daily) are begun around age 35, as well as during pregnancy and nursing, women will start the menopause with thicker, stronger bones. The decline in bone mass that occurs after the menopause (see Chapter 7) will be slower and may not reach the stage where fractures occur. At the time of the menopause or at age 50 (whichever comes first) women would do well to take 1000 mg (one gram) of calcium daily as a supplement, in addition to a diet emphasizing calcium-rich foods (see Chapter 15). Take the calcium pills with meals and in divided doses to enhance absorption — for example, take a 500-mg pill with breakfast and another with dinner.

Many kinds of calcium tablets are currently sold in pharmacies, supermarkets, and health food stores. Most containers list the amount of actual calcium in the tablet; for example, they state that this pill contains 500 mg of calcium. Some brands, however, give the weight of calcium *and* its accompanying compound, such as calcium carbonate, calcium gluconate, or calcium lactate. In general, calcium carbonate is the best buy, as 1000 mg (one gram) of calcium carbonate contains 400 mg of calcium, while 1000 mg of calcium lactate contains only 130 mg of calcium, and 1000 mg of calcium gluconate contains only 100 mg of calcium. Not all brands of calcium tablets dissolve readily in the stomach; if they do not do so you may not absorb the calcium you are taking. Try dropping one of your tablets in a glass of vinegar, stir occasionally and wait about 45 minutes. If the tablet has not dissolved substantially by then you should switch to another brand. Recently calcium has also become available in the form of calcium citrate capsules, which are very easily dissolved and absorbed. If you can find calcium citrate in a natural foods or vitamin store, try it if it is not too expensive.

Prices for calcium tablets vary widely (see accompanying table). You can pay less than $2 or more than $10 per month for a daily gram of calcium. You might consider a reputable mail-order source of supplements such as Bronson Pharmaceuticals (see table).

Vitamin D is also necessary for calcium absorption; it is formed on our skins by sunlight and found in fortified milk products, fish liver oils, and many multivitamin preparations. About 400 IU are needed daily, but much larger doses can be toxic

Name	Amount	Tablets per Gram	Cost per Month
OsCal 500	500 mg per tablet	2	$8 to $10
Generic brands of calcium carbonate	500 mg per tablet	2	$2 to $5
Tums (chewable mint-flavored calcium carbonate)	200 mg per tablet	5	$4 to $5
Bronson* calcium complex	375 mg per tablet	3	$1.32

*Available by mail order from Bronson Pharmaceuticals, 4526 Rinetti Lane, La Cañada, CA 91011.

and should be avoided. Women who do not use milk products should be especially careful to eat other calcium–rich foods and take calcium and vitamin D supplements.

People taking supplementary calcium sometimes worry about developing calcium deposits in their joints or internal organs. This very rare situation occurs when the parathyroid glands, which regulate calcium levels in the body, are overactive, or when too much vitamin D is ingested. It is not a result of taking calcium supplements, which are safe for the vast majority of people. Women with any serious chronic illness or kidney disease should check with their doctors about any supplements.

Kidney stones made of calcium salts occasionally occur, causing pain and medical problems. However, these stones are not the result of increased calcium intake, except in rare cases, for example where large amounts of antacids are being taken for ulcers. They can be the result of a diet too high in protein or salt, and too low in fluids. The excess protein or salt intake causes a greater loss of calcium in the urine, as explained in Chapter 7. During World War II, when meat was very scarce in England and Europe, cases of kidney stone were rarely seen. After the war, when the diet changed to one rich in meat, kidney stones increased in number.

Multivitamins

Multivitamin and multimineral pills are useful if the amounts of vitamins A and D are not too high (not over 15,000 IU of A or 400 IU of D) and if the entire formula is carefully balanced. The advantage of taking such a formula is that you are sure of getting most of the essential nutrients you need daily, which your food may or may not supply. Individuals vary in their requirements for essential nutrients, and a vitamin/mineral supplement in addition to a healthy diet may benefit some people whose needs for a particular nutrient are especially high. Considerable work has gone into determining the minimum amount of vitamins and minerals needed to prevent deficiency diseases; nutrition researchers are now also looking at higher amounts that may optimize health, and at the variable needs of different people.

There are several disadvantages to taking a daily multivitamin/mineral supplement which should be considered. They can be expensive, using money which could more effectively be spent for food and other basic needs. Some people get a false sense of security from supplements, and then subsist on fast food and soft drinks. In so doing, they are overlooking their needs for unrefined carbohydrates and fiber, and ignoring the risks of a diet high in fats and sugars. Finally, some people take huge doses of many vitamins and supplements in a haphazard way, exposing themselves to the risks of toxicity.

I advise middle-aged women to take a balanced multivitamin/mineral tablet daily containing 400 IU of vitamin D (to help with calcium absorption). In addition, I suggest they eat a wide variety of vegetables, fruits, whole grains, and some low-fat animal foods.

In certain circumstances it is an especially good idea to take vitamin and mineral supplements. People on stringent weight control programs often do not eat enough to give themselves the necessary nutrients. People who have lost their appetites because of pain or emotional problems, and patients with chronic diarrhea, alcohol abuse, recent surgery, wounds, burns, or other illness would do well to take daily supplements. Consult with your doctor and a nutritionist to help tailor supplements to your particular needs.

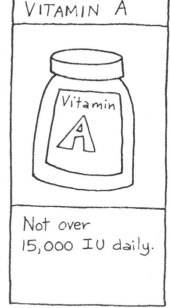

VITAMIN A

Vitamin
A

Not over
15,000 IU daily.

Gerrie had a cabinet full of vitamins, minerals, herbal diuretics, and glandular extracts. At one point she took over 20 pills a day for a few months, and then she abandoned them all in disgust. "I'm not sure what I'm doing or if I notice any difference," she said. "The whole thing is confusing and expensive." Gerrie was anxious because she had had a mastectomy for breast cancer and wanted to avoid a recurrence. Finally her daughter, who was a nurse, sorted out the cabinet and gave her a simpler regimen. "Mom, you should take one multivitamin with minerals, and two calcium pills with a meal. That's 3 pills a day, and I'm going to throw everything else away." Gerrie groaned as she watched all her expensive pills go in the garbage, but she thought her daughter was right. At least she understood now what to take when and why. She felt more secure taking the 3 pills than she had previously felt taking 20.

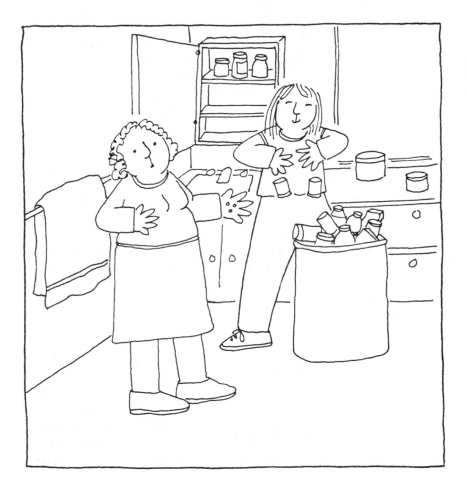

Catherine lived in a halfway house for alcoholics where the food was inexpensive and rather greasy. White bread, lunch meat, canned vegetables, and instant mashed potatoes were the rule. She noticed that her hair was falling out easily, her nails broke, and her energy level was low. She rarely took the time to buy any extra food, but she did get a strong multivitamin and mineral pill which seemed to make a lot of difference in how she felt. "This is crazy," she would say to herself each day as she took her pill, "existing on this terrible food and making it up with vitamins. But right now I have no other choice."

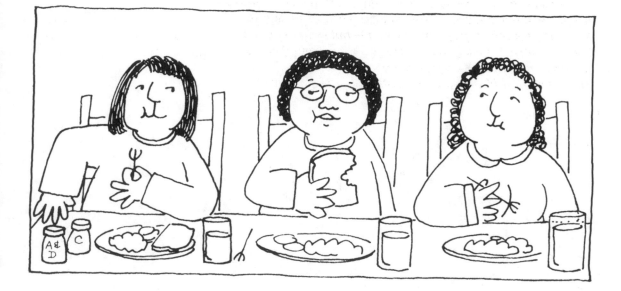

Vitamins/Minerals: Yes or No?

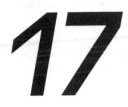

This report points out that the first signs of an epidemic of smoking-related disease among women are now appearing.
— Dr. Julius B. Richmond, U.S. Surgeon General

I am inclined to believe that stopping smoking is very much a personal matter for each one of us. Ultimately, it rests upon a quiet and private decision we make deep within ourselves. Nothing can happen without that decision — not even the most advanced, brilliantly conceived program will work — but everything can happen with it. We each come to that decision in our own way, for our own reasons, and at our own time.
There is no time like the present to start saving your own life.
— Dr. David Geisinger

Smoking — and Quitting

Smoking has been mentioned many times in this book. Everyone knows that smoking is connected to cancer of the lung and other organs, and leads to heart disease and breathing problems in the second half of life. It is less well known that smokers have an earlier menopause, and more problems with brittle bones due to calcium loss (Chapter 7). Smoking is a difficult addiction to overcome, because it is tied in with so many aspects of the smoker's emotional life and daily routines. By mid-life, most smokers have used cigarettes for 20 to 30 years. Yet it is possible to quit — millions of people do so every year. Benefits to your health occur the first day after quitting, and mount over the years. 15 years after you quit, your risk of lung cancer is almost as low as

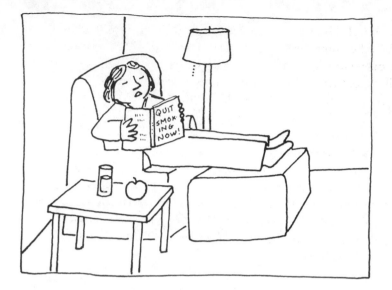

someone who has never smoked. And, as far as menopausal symptoms are concerned, ex-smokers report a decrease in severity of hot flashes and a greater sense of well-being.

If you're a smoker, I strongly urge you to begin the task of quitting by becoming aware of each cigarette you smoke, and figuring out why you need it. Are you smoking out of a need for nicotine, out of habit, or because of emotional needs not connected to a real craving for tobacco? Keep records of your findings. When you are ready, begin to think of yourself as a non-smoker, thereby tuning in to the power of your mind and will to change your life. Get encouragement from non-smoking friends and loved ones, read a book about quitting, join a group, or take a course with other people who are stopping. Programs to help people quit smoking exist in most areas of the country — some, like Smokers Anonymous, are free. Avail yourself of the counsel and experience of other people if support works for you. Once you have made your resolve, set a date to quit within the next 2 weeks. When the day comes, throw away your cigarettes, ashtrays, and lighters. Stay away from other smokers until you are solid in your convictions. Drink lots of water and juices and practice deep breathing. Take yoga classes, which emphasize deep breathing, stretching, relaxation, and health. Nibble on fruit and raw vegetables rather than candy. Eat healthy food, and don't diet at this time. Don't let your fear of weight gain lure you back into smoking! While it's true that most people gain 5 to 10 pounds when they quit smoking, the health benefits of being smoke-free far outweigh the disadvantages of these pounds. Tell yourself you will walk them off as your breathing improves, which it will. Regular exercise, such as a walking program, will help diminish cravings for cigarettes and other withdrawal symptoms.

If you are a heavy smoker and have had severe withdrawal symptoms when trying to quit before, consider asking a doctor to prescribe nicotine gum. Chewing this gum, known as Nicorette, will help you get over the habit of lighting up and will enable your lungs to start healing before you deal with your nicotine addiction. When you feel a strong urge to smoke, you chew a piece of the gum very slowly instead; the nicotine is absorbed into your blood stream through your mouth. You must have quit cigarettes completely before you try the gum. Most people who have benefited from the gum have used it in conjunction with an organized quit-smoking program which explains its use in great detail. Look for one in your community.

Many people who consider giving up tobacco say something like: "I know I should quit, but I just can't seem to do it." Take a moment to analyze this statement. Using the word "should" makes it seem that a higher authority is ordering you to do something, and you can frustrate that higher authority by refusing. Using the word "can't" implies that there is an outside power preventing you from changing your behavior. Actually, of course, it's all inside you — the authority, the power, and the will to bring about successful change.

Harriet had been a smoker for over 30 years. She was a brilliant woman, a rapid and creative thinker who had written several books, and who taught a popular history course at the state university. Cigarettes were her constant companion while she read volumes of material, wrote, corrected students' papers, suffered through faculty meetings, and held court at a local coffee house with the campus intellectuals. She punctuated her thoughts with gestures of hand and cigarette. Close as she was to her cigarettes, Harriet knew they were having drastic effects on her health and stamina. Her doctor had loaned her a book on the health consequences of smoking for women, and Harriet understood that her early and difficult menopause might be related to smoking, as well as her shortness of breath and extreme fatigue. Harriet considered herself a hard-core case in terms of her addiction to tobacco, but she also knew that she was a strong and determined person in most other ways. She decided to go to a live-in stop-smoking program run by the Seventh Day Adventists, in a mountain retreat where there were no cigarettes for sale.

The program was extremely difficult for Harriet, but she appreciated the information, the medical tests, and the group support. She met a 70-year-old man who was attending the program for the third time and intended to succeed this time. By the last day she could walk a mile without stopping or coughing. She set up a buddy system with the older gentleman; they decided to call each other every day to talk about their progress, with S.O.S. calls if they were tempted to smoke. Harriet stayed off cigarettes although it was the hardest thing she had ever done. The next year she organized an elective course on the history of addiction, which was very popular because of her views on the connections between addiction and the profit motive in industrial societies.

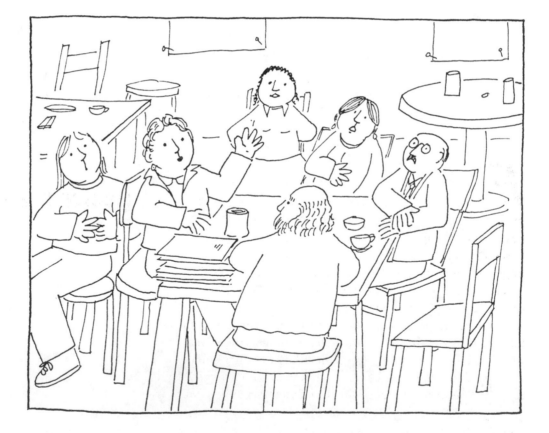

Smoking – and Quitting

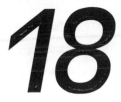

Healing is an equal participation situation — with healer and patient succeeding only if both actively participate in the process.
— *Dr. Mike Samuels*

Health Care

*F*or yearly checkups and for illness, it is important to find a medical practitioner with a positive attitude toward women, health, the menopause, and self-care measures. You may choose to see a gynecologist, a specialist in internal medicine or a family or general practitioner. Alternatively, you may go to a clinic where you see one of the types of doctors just mentioned or a physician's assistant or nurse practitioner.* It is important that any such health professional be interested in women's medicine, take the time to listen to your problems and questions, and perform a thorough yearly exam including a check of blood pressure, heart and lungs, breasts, abdomen, pelvic organs, and rectum. Your practitioner should teach you to examine your own

---

* Physician's assistants and nurse practitioners are health professionals trained to assess health and illness, counsel on health practices, and prescribe certain medicines under the supervision of a doctor. They are providing high-quality women's health care in many areas.

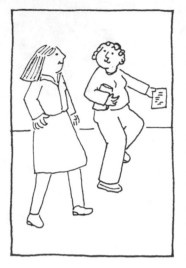

breasts. She or he should also be able to advise you on questions concerning drugs, alcohol, smoking, exercise, nutrition and stress. A medical practitioner with an open mind about the benefits and risks of estrogen therapy will enable women to choose what is best for them in this area.

Patients, for their part, should be as clear as possible about their problems, and should keep records of their symptoms. You should say that you want information, counseling, physical therapy, or nutritional advice — unless medicine or surgery are absolutely necessary. It is a good idea to write out your questions before an appointment, so you are sure to get them answered. Go to your appointment with a friend who will be your advocate if you are anxious. Feel free to go to another doctor for a second opinion if any treatment is suggested that seems unnecessary to you.

Doctors who take a positive view of the menopause, and do not routinely view ill health and pain as inevitable parts of aging, can help women with mid-life problems. However, much of medical education has a disease orientation which tends to make doctors pessimistic. Consider, for example, this amazingly negative quote from a recent medical textbook summarizing the latest facts in gynecology:

Although menopause, the last menstrual period, is just a single point in the protracted unfolding of the climacteric, only the most stoic, objective and rationally composed human can dismiss it as a minor physiologic event. For most women, it signals an end to the known, the accustomed, and the expected, and the beginning of an era of insidiously diminishing competence, leading irretrievably to aging and death. Add to this gloomy prospect the almost obsessive cultish pursuit of youthful sexual femininity that our society espouses, and one can only wonder why more post-menopausal women do not complicate their physiologic deficits with great emotional burdens.

— Precis II: An Update in Obstetrics and Gynecology,
The American College of Obstetricians and Gynecologists, 1981, page 141.

When negative value judgments like this are propounded as facts, it's not surprising that many doctors continue to over-medicate older women. Instead of viewing low estrogen levels as nature's norm in the post-reproductive years, doctors may say that a woman's vaginal tissues are "estrogen starved," or showing signs of "senile vaginitis." Such attitudes on the part of the doctor can be much more painful than the vaginal problem itself. Hence, it is important for women to find doctors with positive views of the aging process, which is why the newly forming network of menopause clinics in women's health centers is so valuable.

The same careful approach is needed in choosing a counselor for emotional and psychological help. Mid-life women should look for a well-trained person (such as a social worker, licensed counselor, psychologist, or psychiatrist) with whom it is comfortable to talk. Look for someone who helps clients with emotional pain and encourages personal growth. Group therapy and mid-life self-help groups are also available in some areas. This kind of counseling is more helpful for most people than the kind which routinely uses tranquilizers or anti-depressants. As a rule, take as few drugs of any kind as possible, and make sure your doctor knows all the drugs you are taking.

Bernice went to Dr. Williams because of soreness with intercourse. She was nervous about the visit because she had not seen him in two years, and she feared he would pressure her to take post-menopausal estrogens as he did with most of his patients. Bernice was also anxious because she had met a new man this year, 5 years after her divorce, and she wasn't sure how Dr. Williams would react to her having an affair. She got undressed and, lying on the examining table, waited for him to arrive. When he did a pelvic exam, Dr. Williams remarked that she had a bad case of "senile vaginal atrophy" and he pointed out the characteristics of the problem to a medical student who was working with him. Bernice felt angry and embarrassed by this episode. She accepted Dr. William's prescription for estrogen tablets in order to get out of his office as quickly as possible. Once home, she cried, punched her pillow, and decided she had to find another doctor.

She found out that a women's center in a nearby city had opened a special service for mid-life women. Bernice went there the next week and had quite a different experience. She was given some interesting pamphlets on the menopause, sex, aging, and the pros and cons of estrogen therapy. In a relaxed discussion with a nurse practitioner, she found out that she could use a small amount of estrogen cream twice a week and not take pills for her problem of soreness. Above all, she found out that the physical examination did not have to be painful or embarrassing, but could be informative and reassuring. She came away feeling more self-confident and hopeful about her new love affair.

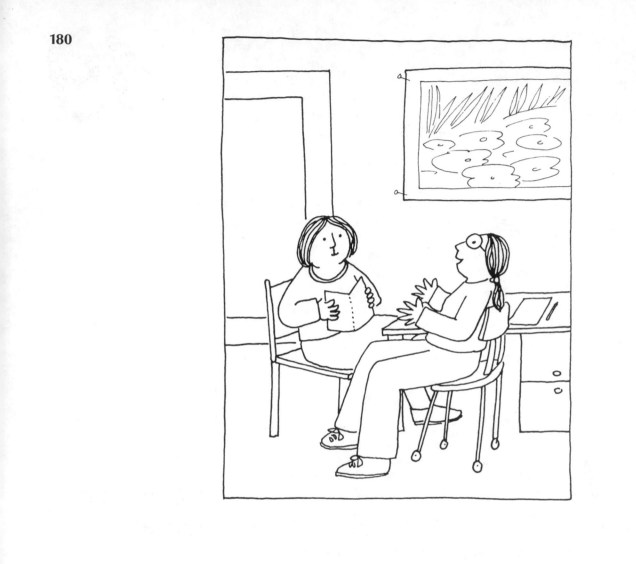

Health Care

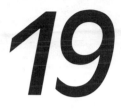

I have described numerous paths to the goal of post-menopausal zest, and proposed a positive view of ourselves in mid-life. Staying connected to the world; relaxation, exercise, nutrition, supplements; not smoking; and finding good health care — each is an important part of every day we live.

In and after the menopausal years, women have certain special needs, problems, and advantages. Their special needs are for more calcium, more exercise, and more attention to healthful, balanced living. Their special problems are those of hot flashes, brittle bones, and vaginal soreness with intercourse. Their special advantages are that the period of life after the menopause is smoother — no more premenstrual tension, hormonal mood swings, pelvic aching, or menstrual problems. No more concerns about birth control. Daily life seems to many women to have more balance and steadiness. Post-menopausal zest can become a reality!

Summing It All Up!

In China, the sixtieth birthday is considered a momentous event, a time when the family gathers to celebrate the status and wisdom of the elder. Other societies which revere age have special positions for older women which acknowledge their worth and power. Aging is seen as a gain in wisdom and not just a loss of youth. Interestingly enough, in these societies, the menopause is not viewed as a negative event, but as a time when women rise in social status and enjoy more privileges.

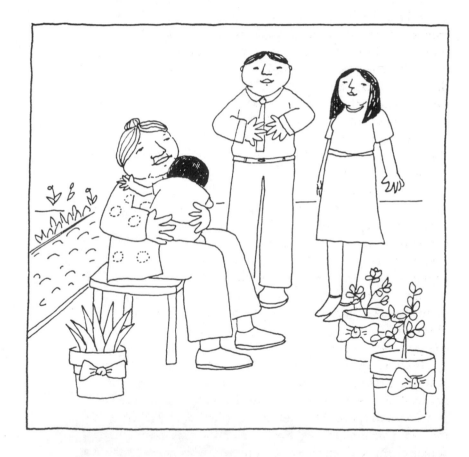

Can this be so in our society? Yes, if we make it so. Although our culture has glorified youth, especially in women, this emphasis is changing. As birthrates stay low and the life span increases, we find an increasing proportion of our citizens in middle- and old-age groups. This phenomenon has been called the "graying of America." Mid-life and older people are becoming a stronger social and political force. Two other factors are also at work — the philosophy of personhood and the women's movement.

The philosophy of personhood is an emerging view in our culture; it holds that each person is not only equal but unique, and should develop her or his potential, regardless of age, sex, or ethnic group. We can go back to school in our 50s, take up new interests in our 60s, and change our names or our sexual orientations. This view of life allows mid-life women to free themselves from old stereotypes and gain a sense of self-worth. The women's movement does the same thing, and encourages women to use their conviction of equality and power in the world around them — at work, at home, and in their communities and nations. Once women achieve feelings of real self-worth, regardless of age or appearance, they will see middle age or menopause not as a tragedy, but as a time of accumulated wisdom and experience. They can see the second half of life building on the first half and developing from it in new ways.

I have discussed the special needs and problems of mid-life in some detail. But what *you* do with post-menopausal zest is the next chapter, for you to write for yourself. Some women need to concentrate on survival or sanity in this difficult world. Others want to develop themselves in new ways they have not yet explored. Some women will become strong figures in their families; others will be more active in their communities once family responsibilities decrease. Some will use their creativity for the good of the planet, which desperately needs more female energy to heal its rifts.

Need a model? Notice how many of the Nobel Prizes for peace have recently gone to women: Alva Myrdal of Sweden for her work on disarmament, Mother Teresa of Calcutta for her work with the poor, Mairead Corrigan and Betty Williams of Northern Ireland for their work to stop the fighting in their country. Think about Millicent Fenwick, who served in the U.S senate in her 70s and then went to work on world food problems. All these women have used the special wisdom and experience of being female to inspire their action in the world.

Meredith spoke of her mid-life changes very emphatically. "I began to know myself in a new way after the children left home and I turned 50. I saw that my life was limited and yet unlimited at the same time. Limited in that I wouldn't live forever. Unlimited in that I could really be myself for the first time in many years. I decided to put my energies into the political work that had always interested me, and within two years I was running for city councilwoman. I feel I can take all my talents in working with and for people, and use them in a larger way in politics. I'd like to see a lot more women, especially older women, getting into community leadership. They've got a lot of wisdom to share.

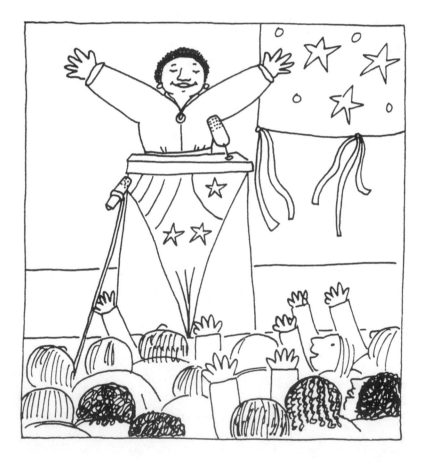

Adoption

Canape, C. *Adoption: Parenthood without Pregnancy.* Henry Holt,
New York, 1986. The author's experiences with adoption,
including excellent appendices of adoption agencies and
support groups across the country.

Martin, C. *Beating the Adoption Game.* Oak Tree Press, San
Diego, 1980. A complete book about adoption, including a
section on accelerating the process through private adoptions.
Very good on the practical and psychological aspects of
adoption.

Cancer

Doll, R., and Peto, R. *The Causes of Cancer.* Oxford University
Press, New York, 1981. A detailed scientific discussion of the
avoidable risks of cancer in the U.S. today, including tobacco,
alcohol, diet, reproductive and sexual behavior, and environmental factors.

Simonton, O. C., et al. *Getting Well Again.* J. P. Tarcher, Los
Angeles, 1978. A book about the uses of relaxation and
imagery to assist in the healing of cancer, as an adjunct to
surgery, radiation, and chemotherapy. The authors stress that
imagery is not to be relied on by itself to cure cancer, but that
it should be used in addition to more proven treatments.

**Suggestions
for Further
Reading**

Spletter, M. *A Woman's Choice; New Options in the Treatment of Breast Cancer.* Beacon Press, Boston, 1982. A clear and thorough explanation of breast cancer and its treatment options by a science writer who has had the disease. She explores the medical, psychological, and cosmetic facets of mastectomy and reconstructive surgery.

Subak-Sharpe, G. *Overcoming Breast Cancer.* Doubleday & Co., New York, 1987. A thorough discussion of breast cancer and its current treatments written by doctors for the general public. Includes material on the dietary approach to breast cancer prevention.

Exercise

Anderson, B. *Stretching.* Shelter Publications, P.O. Box 279, Bolinas, CA 94924, 1980. A guide to stretching exercises for every part of the body, emphasizing ease and good feelings. Stretching programs for all sports.

Cooper, K. H. *The Aerobics Way.* M. Evans & Co., New York, 1977. An explanation of the benefits of vigorous exercise, followed by detailed plans for gradual conditioning for all age groups in a variety of activities (walking, jogging, cycling, swimming, racquet sports, stationary bicycling, stair climbing, rope skipping). Includes plans for the very obese and for people who have had coronary bypass surgery.

Hittleman, R. *Richard Hittleman's Yoga: 28-Day Exercise Plan.* Bantam Books, New York, 1969. A systematic beginner's guide to yoga postures with illustrations of each exercise. Gently leads into flexibility and more peace of mind.

Root, L., et al. *Oh, My Aching Back.* Signet, New York, 1975. An excellent book on back problems with explanations of their causes, and a series of back exercises to promote flexibility and strength and to prevent pain.

Women's Health Problems

Hasselbring, B., Greenwood, S., et al. *The Medical Self-Care Book of Women's Health.* Doubleday & Co., New York, 1987. A resource book on many women's health problems, with an emphasis on what you can do to prevent illness and take care of yourself. Coauthored by Sadja Greenwood, author of *Menopause Naturally.*

Stewart, F., et al. *Understanding Your Body: Every Woman's Guide to* **187**
Gynecology and Health. Bantam Books, New York, 1987. An
excellent, comprehensive guide to women's health,
emphasizing prevention as well as treatment.

Menopause

Budoff, P. W., *No More Hot Flashes and Other Good News.* G.P.
Putnam's Sons, New York, 1983. A well researched book by
a woman physician on menopause, osteoporosis, breast and
ovarian cancer, urinary incontinence and birth control in
mid-life. Emphasizes hormone replacement therapy.

Cutler, W. B., et al. *Menopause, A Guide for Women and the Men
Who Love Them.* W.W. Norton & Company, New York,
1983. A scholarly book on menopausal problems favoring
hormone use, and providing a thorough discussion of its
benefits and risks.

Downing, C. *Journey through Menopause — A Personal Rite of
Passage.* Crossroads Publishing Co., New York, 1987. In this
tale of a journey through menopause and around the world,
the author finds meanings in mythology, poetry, and travel
for "the change of life," seen as a journey of the soul.

Voda, A. M., Dinnerstein, M., O'Donnell, S. R., editors.
Changing Perspective on Menopause. University of Texas Press,
Austin, 1982. A collection of essays by contemporary scholars
on the menopause, from an anthropologic, literary, psychological, and physiological perspective. Excellent original
material.

Voda, A. M., *Menopause, Me and You.* Booklet available by
writing to Dr. Ann Voda, College of Nursing, 25 South
Medical Drive, Salt Lake City, Utah 84112. Excellent information on hot flashes and other aspects of menopause, not
oriented to hormone use.

Nutrition

Brody, J. *Jane Brody's Good Food Book.* Bantam Books, Inc., New
York, 1987. A wonderful source book on nutrition and
healthy foods, with recipes low in fat and salt, written by a
New York Times science writer.

Lappé, F. M. *Diet for a Small Planet:* 10th Anniversary Edition. Ballantine Books, New York, 1982. The famous book on the importance of a plant-based diet to individual health and world food shortages, revised and updated. Simplified and delicious recipes.

Robertson, L., et al. *The New Laurel's Kitchen, A Handbook for Vegetarian Cookery and Nutrition.* Ten Speed Press, Berkeley, CA, 1986. Excellent recipes, very health conscious, followed by a comprehensive and updated nutrition section.

Shulman, M. R. *Fast Vegetarian Feasts: The Revised Edition with Fish.* Doubleday and Co., New York, 1986. Healthy and delicious recipes, low in fat and salt, prepared in 45 minutes or less.

Worthington-Roberts, B. S. *Contemporary Developments in Nutrition.* C. V. Mosby, St. Louis, 1981. A detailed, scientific textbook on nutrition with a health-oriented perspective.

Osteoporosis

Fardon, D. F. *Osteoporosis: Your Head Start on the Prevention and Treatment of Brittle Bones.* Macmillan Publishing Co., New York, 1985. An informative book on osteoporosis, written by an orthopedic surgeon.

Notelovitz, M., et al. *Stand Tall: The Informed Women's Guide to Preventing Osteoporosis.* Triad Publishing Company, P.O. Box 13096, Gainesville, FL 32604, 1982. An exceedingly informative book about osteoporosis, its causes, and measures to prevent it.

Sexuality

Barbach, L., et al. *Shared Intimacies: Women's Sexual Experiences.* Anchor Press/Doubleday, Garden City, New York, 1980. An excellent book of interviews with women of all ages, about their sexual experiences and commentary by the authors, both women and sex therapists. Interesting, diverse material on sex in the menopause and beyond.

Blank, J. *Good Vibrations: Mail Order Catalog,* 3492 22nd St., San Francisco, CA 94110. A woman-owned business devoted to sexual pleasure and information. The catalog lists vibrators, sex toys, condoms, and many good books relating to women's sexual problems and pleasures. Highly recommended.

Ferguson, T. *The Smoker's Book of Health*. G. P. Putnam's Sons, New York, 1987. A very practical guide for smokers on how to lower your risks even while smoking, and how to quit when you're ready, written by a physician.

Gahagan, D. *Switch Down and Quit*. Ten Speed Press, Berkeley, CA, 1987. A very savvy book on nicotine addiction and how to overcome it, and on the role of cigarette advertising in maintaining your addiction.

Geisinger, D. *Kicking It*. Signet, New American Library, New York, 1980. An excellent book on how to quit smoking by a skillful psychologist.

U.S. Surgeon General. *The Health Consequences of Smoking for Women*. U.S. Department of Health and Human Services, Public Health Service, 1980. A comprehensive analysis of the effects of smoking on women's health, including pregnancy, cancer, the menopause, osteoporosis, ovarian function, and other topics.

Stress and Relaxation

Benson, H. *The Relaxation Response*. Avon, New York, 1975. An excellent short book by a Harvard physician on how and why to make a daily habit of relaxation.

Friedman, M., and Rosenman, R. H., *Type A Behavior and Your Heart*. Fawcett Publications, Greenwich, CT, 1974. The original book about the effects of behavior on heart disease, with an excellent discussion of the stress derived from a chronic sense of time urgency. Many practical ways to live more slowly and gently are described.

Nuernberger, P. *Freedom from Stress, a Holistic Approach*. Himalayan International Institute of Yoga Science and Philosophy, Honesdale, PA, 1981. A remarkable book explaining the basics of the central nervous system, the problems of stress, and the reasons and ways that meditation can be helpful.

Ornish, D. *Stress, Diet and Your Heart*. New American Library/ Signet, New York, 1984. A program of stress reduction and nutrition to prevent or reverse heart disease, by one of the first doctors to study and demonstrate that such a program is effective. The relaxation exercises are widely applicable.

Newsletters on Health Topics and Aging

A Friend Indeed. P.O. Box 9, NGD Station, Montreal H4A 3P4, Canada. A lively, informative, sharing newsletter, exploring menopause as mythology, biology, and feelings.

Hot Flash: Newsletter for Midlife and Older Women. Box 816, Stony Brook, NY 11790-0609. A newsletter devoted to promoting post-menopausal zest by giving information on the health, mental needs, and resources of older women.

Medical Self Care. P.O. Box 717, Inverness, CA 94937. A quarterly magazine on all aspects of health, self-care, and consumer-oriented medicine. Good layout, informal, and understandable. Women's health column is written by Dr. Sadja Greenwood, the author of this book.

Network. National Gray Panther Newsletter, 3635 Chestnut Street, Philadelphia, PA 19104. A newsletter published every other month discussing issues related to aging, health care, political and social action, and activities of local chapters.

Nutrition Action Healthletter. Center for Science in the Public Interest, 1501 16th Street, NW, Washington, D.C. 20036. A monthly magazine on practical nutritional information and the political battles for consumer education about food and health. Witty, well illustrated, and easy to read.

Volcano Press publishes titles of special interest to women:

_____ **Menopause, Naturally: Preparing for the Second Half of Life**, $11.95
Revised, by Sadja Greenwood, M.D., M.P.H.

_____ **The Infertility Book: A Comprehensive Medical and Emotional** $12.00
Guide by Carla Harkness. Examines medical, emotional, legal,
financial, and ethical issues; discusses adoption, surrogate mothering
and child-free living.

_____ **Goddesses** by Mayumi Oda. Drawing her full color images from old $14.95
Japanese prints, Oda transforms traditional Buddhist gods into their
joyous female counter-parts. Accompanied by a lyrical, political
autobiography.

_____ **Period** by JoaAnn Gardner-Loulan, Bonnie Lopez, and Marcia $ 9.95
Quackenbush. A friendly, supportive book on menstruation, written
and illustrated in a reassuring, informative way for girls and their
parents.

_____ **Período: Libro para chicas sobre la menstruación.** Spanish edition $ 7.00
of Period. (See above).

_____ **El lenguaje de la sexualidad para la mujer y la pareja.** $11.00
by Yael Fischman, Ph.D. Informed, comprehensive answers to
frequently asked questions about sexuality by a Latina therapist.
In Spanish.

_____ **Conspiracy of Silence: The Trauma of Incest** by Sandra Butler. $11.95
Thoroughly researched and well documented, while encouraging the
individual to understand and resolve personal issues.

_____ **Battered Wives** by Del Martin. The first and still the best introduction $11.95
to the problem of abuse.

_____ **Learning to Live Without Violence: A Handbook for Men,** $11.95
Updated by Daniel J. Sonkin, Ph.D. and Michael Durphy, M.D. A
14-week program providing batterers with techniques for redirecting
their anger and developing healthier relationships.

Buy these books through your local bookstore, or order directly from:

Volcano Press, P.O. Box 270 MN, Volcano, CA 95689
Tel: (209) 296-3445   Telex: 650-3491755   Fax: (209) 296-4515

Please send me the books I have checked above. I am enclosing _____ which includes $3.50
postage and handling for the first book ordered, and $1.00 for additional titles.

California state residents please add 6% sales tax.

Name _____
Address _____
City _____   State/Zip _____

_____ Please send me your catalog.

Volcano Press books are available at special quantity discounts for bulk purchases, for professional counseling, educational, fundraising or premium use.

For details, write or telephone:

Volcano Press, Inc., P.O. Box 270, Volcano, California 95689 U.S.A. (209) 296-3445.